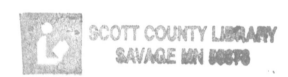

SCOTT COUNTY LIBRARY
SAVAGE MN 55378

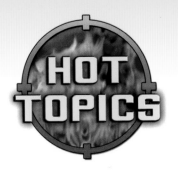

Health Care

by Debra A. Miller

LUCENT BOOKS
A part of Gale, Cengage Learning

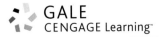
GALE
CENGAGE Learning™

Detroit • New York • San Francisco • New Haven, Conn • Waterville, Maine • London

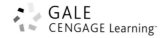

© 2011 Gale, Cengage Learning

ALL RIGHTS RESERVED. No part of this work covered by the copyright herein may be reproduced, transmitted, stored, or used in any form or by any means graphic, electronic, or mechanical, including but not limited to photo-copying, recording, scanning, digitizing, taping, Web distribution, information networks, or information storage and retrieval systems, except as permit-ted under Section 107 or 108 of the 1976 United States Copyright Act, with-out the prior written permission of the publisher.

Every effort has been made to trace the owners of copyrighted material.

LIBRARY OF CONGRESS CATALOGING-IN-PUBLICATION DATA

Miller, Debra A.
  Health care / by Debra A. Miller.
     p. cm. -- (Hot topics)
  Includes bibliographical references and index.
  ISBN 978-1-4205-0568-9 (hardcover)
  1. Medical care--United States--Popular works. 2. Health care reform--
United States--Popular works. 3. Medical care--Popular works. I. Title.
  RA395.A3M52 2011
  362.1'0425--dc22

                                                              2010041798

Lucent Books
27500 Drake Rd.
Farmington Hills, MI 48331

ISBN-13: 978-1-4205-0568-9
ISBN-10: 1-4205-0568-8

Printed in the United States of America
1 2 3 4 5 6 7 15 14 13 12 11

Printed by Bang Printing, Brainerd, MN, 1st Ptg., 02/2011

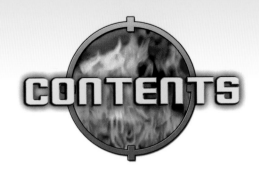

CONTENTS

FOREWORD 4

INTRODUCTION 6
The Uninsured in America

CHAPTER 1 11
America's Health Care System

CHAPTER 2 27
The Debate About Health Care Reform

CHAPTER 3 43
Health Care Systems in Other Countries

CHAPTER 4 59
The Patient Protection and Affordable Care Act

CHAPTER 5 75
The Future of U.S. Health Care

NOTES 91

DISCUSSION QUESTIONS 97

ORGANIZATIONS TO CONTACT 99

FOR MORE INFORMATION 103

INDEX 107

PICTURE CREDITS 111

ABOUT THE AUTHOR 112

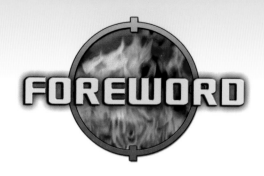

FOREWORD

Young people today are bombarded with information. Aside from traditional sources such as newspapers, television, and the radio, they are inundated with a nearly continuous stream of data from electronic media. They send and receive e-mails and instant messages, read and write online "blogs," participate in chat rooms and forums, and surf the Web for hours. This trend is likely to continue. As Patricia Senn Breivik, the former dean of university libraries at Wayne State University in Detroit, has stated, "Information overload will only increase in the future. By 2020, for example, the available body of information is expected to double every 73 days! How will these students find the information they need in this coming tidal wave of information?"

Ironically, this overabundance of information can actually impede efforts to understand complex issues. Whether the topic is abortion, the death penalty, gay rights, or obesity, the deluge of fact and opinion that floods the print and electronic media is overwhelming. The news media report the results of polls and studies that contradict one another. Cable news shows, talk radio programs, and newspaper editorials promote narrow viewpoints and omit facts that challenge their own political biases. The World Wide Web is an electronic minefield where legitimate scholars compete with the postings of ordinary citizens who may or may not be well-informed or capable of reasoned argument. At times, strongly worded testimonials and opinion pieces both in print and electronic media are presented as factual accounts.

Conflicting quotes and statistics can confuse even the most diligent researchers. A good example of this is the question of whether or not the death penalty deters crime. For instance, one study found that murders decreased by nearly one-third when the death penalty was reinstated in New York in 1995. Death penalty supporters cite this finding to support their argument that the existence of the death penalty deters criminals from committing murder. However, another study found that states without the death penalty have murder rates below the national average. This study is cited by opponents of capital punishment, who reject the claim that the death penalty deters murder. Students need context and clear, informed discussion if they are to think critically and make informed decisions.

The Hot Topics series is designed to help young people wade through the glut of fact, opinion, and rhetoric so that they can think critically about controversial issues. Only by reading and thinking critically will they be able to formulate a viewpoint that is not simply the parroted views of others. Each volume of the series focuses on one of today's most pressing social issues and provides a balanced overview of the topic. Carefully crafted narrative, fully documented primary and secondary source quotes, informative sidebars, and study questions all provide excellent starting points for research and discussion. Full-color photographs and charts enhance all volumes in the series. With its many useful features, the Hot Topics series is a valuable resource for young people struggling to understand the pressing issues of the modern era.

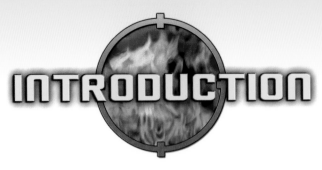

INTRODUCTION

THE UNINSURED IN AMERICA

The U.S. health care system has often been called the best in the world. It develops and implements the newest medical technologies, boasts world-class facilities and highly trained doctors, and is capable of providing prompt and cutting-edge patient care. The United States also spends more than any other country on health care, both per capita (per person) and in terms of total health expenditures as a percentage of the gross domestic product (GDP)—the country's total economic output. Yet despite these positives, the United States consistently scores at or near the bottom when its health care system is compared with those in other developed countries on issues such as quality, efficiency, and effectiveness of care. In fact, according to every independent study, the United States has the highest rates of infant mortality, the lowest levels of life expectancy, and the largest number of people without health insurance coverage of almost any other developed nation. As Steffie Woolhandler, a professor of medicine at Harvard Medical School and cofounder of Physicians for a National Health Program, puts it, "The U.S. has . . . arguably the worst [health care system] in the developed world."[1]

The most glaring problem with U.S. health care, according to the research, is the high number of uninsured people. In other developed countries, almost everyone is covered by health insurance, typically under some type of government-regulated or government-run program. In the United States, however, health insurance is an employer-based, privately operated system, and a growing segment of the population has no insurance coverage. In fact, according to a September 2009 report from the U.S. Census Bureau, 46.3 million Americans, or roughly 15 percent of the total population, had no health insurance in 2008, the last year for which statistics are available. Contrary to what logic might suggest, this uninsured population is not made up largely of poor, aged, or unemployed people. According to the Census Bureau, nearly all the uninsured are under age 65, most earn more than $25,000 per year (20 percent had incomes above $50,000), and only about 9.9 percent are children. This is because the elderly, the poor, and many children are now covered by government health programs such as Medicare, Medicaid, and the State Children's Health Insurance Program. Moreover, 82.8 percent of the nonelderly uninsured live in fami-

Volunteer dentists work on patients at a free clinic in Los Angeles. Free clinics have been staged all over the country in an effort to give health care to millions of uninsured Americans.

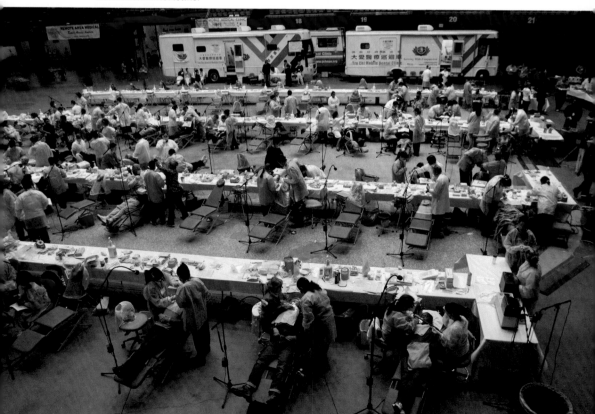

lies where the head of household works. And even though many large employers in the United States provide health insurance as an employee benefit, one in five of the uninsured works in a large company (defined as a firm with five hundred or more employees) yet does not receive health benefits.

Clear racial, ethnic, and immigration status trends are evident in the uninsured statistics, however. In 2008, 30.7 percent of Hispanics were uninsured, as were 19.1 percent of African Americans, 17.6 of Asians, and 31.7 percent of American Indians and Alaska Natives, compared with a 10.8 percent uninsured rate for whites. As a report from the nonprofit Robert Woods Johnson Foundation explains, "Relative to their numbers in the overall population, members of racial and ethnic minority groups make up a disproportionate share of the uninsured population."[2] Also, according to Census Bureau estimates, 33.5 percent of the uninsured are immigrants, with noncitizens making up 18 percent of this immigrant population. The number of illegal immigrants who are uninsured, however, is not known.

The main reason for the lack of insurance, many experts say, is affordability; health insurance costs have been rising rapidly since the 1960s. Although some young, healthy people choose to go without insurance because they feel they are invincible, increasing numbers of Americans want health insurance but just cannot afford it. The luckiest are people who get health insurance from their employers as part of their salary package, but rising premium costs have caused many employers to drop or cut back on health insurance in recent years. That leaves noncovered employees, along with the self-employed, to fend for themselves in the individual insurance policy market, where they have little negotiating power and face large premiums. In fact, even those who are able to afford insurance may not be granted coverage by insurers because they have preexisting medical conditions—that is, conditions diagnosed before patients apply for insurance. Many others—some estimates say 25 million—purchase policies but are still underinsured. In the case of a serious medical event, their insurance would pay for only part of their health expenses, not only because of large co-pays (what the patient pays in addition to insurance) and deductibles but also because

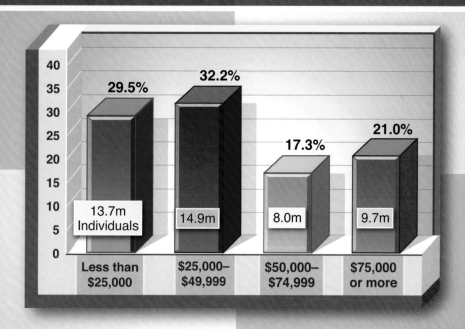

Uninsured Americans by Household Income, 2008

29.5%	32.2%	17.3%	21.0%
13.7m Individuals	14.9m	8.0m	9.7m
Less than $25,000	$25,000–$49,999	$50,000–$74,999	$75,000 or more

Taken from: U.S. Census Bureau.

of annual or lifetime limits in their policies. Counting both the uninsured and the underinsured, Jonathan Cohn, author of a recent book about health care, estimates that "almost one fourth of Americans don't have adequate health benefits."[3]

According to health experts, this lack of adequate health insurance has far-reaching consequences for families, communities, and U.S. society. According to the National Institute of Medicine (IOM), an independent health research group in the National Academy of Sciences, people without health insurance experience poorer health, die sooner, and are more likely to go bankrupt as a result of health costs than those who are insured—all tragic results for families and loved ones. A large number of uninsured citizens also reduces the financial stability of local hospitals and medical providers, decreasing access and quality of care for everyone in the community. According to many researchers, societal costs are incurred as well, in terms of reduced work productivity, taxpayer dollars spent on emergency and government-subsidized care, and loss of public confidence in American ideals of fairness and equality.

This ever-worsening state of affairs has been the catalyst for repeated efforts to enact health care reform in the United States. Most recently, in March 2010, the U.S. Congress passed the Patient Protection and Affordable Care Act (PPACA or ACA), a landmark health care reform law championed by President Barack Obama. The ACA, however, is the culmination of a long health care journey for the United States that began early in the nineteenth century, and people have differing views about whether it will improve care or cut costs.

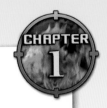

AMERICA'S HEALTH CARE SYSTEM

The modern medical care considered the norm today is actually a fairly new phenomenon in America. During colonial and revolutionary times, medicine was largely a medieval art with virtually no scientific basis. Traditional medical practitioners at this time believed that the body contained four "humors"—blood (fire), phlegm (earth), black bile (water), and yellow bile (air)—and that the work of physicians was to maintain a balance among these influences. To accomplish this, doctors largely relied on a limited supply of herbs and drugs, some of which (such as mercury) were quite toxic. Other early medical treatments included bleedings (withdrawing sometimes considerable amounts of blood from sick patients) and purgings (using laxatives, diuretics, or medicines to make patients vomit or otherwise excrete wastes)—practices which many times were harmful rather than helpful to patients. Medical schools did not exist at this time, and medical training largely consisted of working as an apprentice to an existing practitioner. People who got sick generally paid out of pocket for their medical treatments, but costs were quite low, perhaps because results were often negative.

During the second half of the nineteenth century, however, advances in biology and chemistry helped medical doctors better understand the human body, incorporating principles of modern science into the practice of medicine. Sanitation became an important method of preventing infection, more effective treatments for diseases and injuries were developed, and surgical techniques were refined. In 1847 the American Medical Association (AMA) was founded to create professional standards for

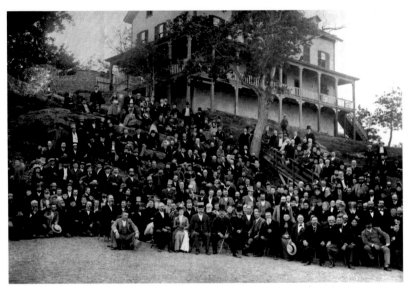

Members of the American Medical Association meet in Rhode Island in 1889. Founded in 1847, the AMA created professional standards for doctors and set minimum educational requirements.

doctors and set minimum educational requirements. Thereafter, numerous medical colleges were established, medical research expanded, and hospitals were built across the nation. During the twentieth century, the state of medical care and technologies developed even more. However, as medicine became more effective, the cost of care rose, and a system of health insurance gradually developed to spread the risks and help people pay for this more advanced health care.

Early Health Insurance Programs

According to Cohn, the modern era of medicine in the United States began in the 1920s. Around this time, the cost of medical care had exploded to the point that it became unaffordable to many Americans. When the U.S. and world economy began to sink into the Great Depression in the late 1920s, the situation only worsened. As Cohn explains, "The average cost of a week in the hospital began to exceed what the majority of Americans earned in a month, making illness a scary financial proposition for even the thriftiest middle class households—and forcing many people to skip medical care altogether."[4]

To address this problem, several private philanthropic foundations in 1927 established the Committee on the Costs of Medical Care (CCMC) to study the health care crisis and report on possible solutions. The committee's final report in October 1932 recommended the creation of health insurance for medical care. The report explained that this made sense because health expenses tend to be concentrated on people with serious medical conditions, and since everyone faced the prospect of some type of serious medical crisis during his or her lifetime, health costs could be reduced if collective systems were developed to insure against serious illness.

One of the first efforts to provide prepaid health care, however, was initiated by Baylor Hospital in Dallas, Texas, in 1929, even before the CCMC's report was released. The hospital's administrator, who had a background working with public schools, offered to provide up to twenty days of hospital care

By 1930 the average cost of a week in the hospital exceeded what most Americans earned in a month. Many people were forced to skip any kind of medical care.

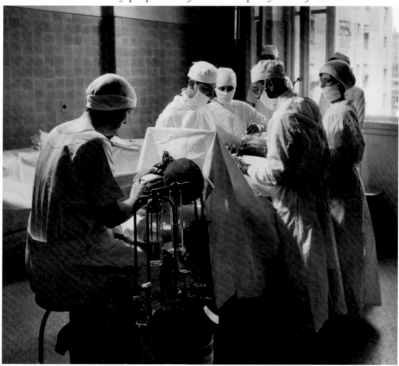

for local teachers if at least three-quarters of the teachers in the region agreed to be part of the plan. The Baylor plan worked, covering the hospital costs of about fifteen hundred teachers for a monthly premium of about fifty cents. News of the success of this early insurance plan spread around the country to other hospitals and eventually evolved into a national system called Blue Cross.

ADVANCEMENTS IN MEDICINE

"Scientific research and development have produced a burgeoning array of medications, medical procedures, and instruments, along with a growing understanding of the basic elements of human health, all of which have made dramatic contributions to the length and quality of life."—George P. Shultz, a former U.S. secretary of state during the Ronald Reagan administration and currently a fellow at the conservative think tank the Hoover Institution.

George P. Shultz and John B. Shoven, *Putting Our House in Order: A Guide to Social Security and Health Care Reform.* New York: W.W. Norton, 2008, p. 126.

The early Blue Cross insurers were typically private nonprofits created to cover large groups of employees (or sometimes groups of people affiliated with fraternal societies such as the Elks Club) because they needed a pool large enough to spread the risks. Even though they were private entities, these early insurers provided a public benefit. They charged everyone the same premium regardless of age, sex, or preexisting conditions—a system called community rate—and many also provided some form of insurance to individuals who agreed to pay their premiums. With no pressure to produce profits, premiums were kept low, supported only by government tax deductions. As Cohn explains, Blue Cross thus "resemble[d] social insurance—a protection scheme in which healthy people subsidized the costs of the sick, precisely as the Committee on the Cost of Medicine had recommended in 1932."[5]

An Employer-Based Health Insurance System

The entrance of America into World War II in the 1940s helped to establish a uniquely American system of employer-based health insurance. When the government imposed wage controls on employers during the war, many employers began offering health insurance as an employee benefit. The United States at that time suffered from a very tight labor market, since many workers were in active duty with the armed forces, and health insurance was one of the few incentives employers could offer

The Modern Medicare System

Medicare has changed somewhat since its enactment in 1965. Today, Medicare still has the original Parts A and B, but it also has Part C and Part D. With certain exceptions, anyone who has been a legal resident of the United States for five years and who is sixty-five years old or older is eligible for Medicare insurance, and there is no premium if the individual or his or her spouse has paid into the system for a minimum of ten years. After a deductible of $1,068, Medicare Part A pays for inpatient care in hospitals, some short-term care at a skilled nursing facility or hospice, as well as some home health care services. However, Medicare only pays in full for hospital stays up to 60 days; after that patients must pay coinsurance, and for hospital stays longer than 150 days, Medicare pays nothing. Similarly, Medicare Part B helps cover doctor services and out-patient care, plus some preventive services, but generally this help is limited to 80 percent of the Medicare-approved amount for covered services (many people purchase private insurance to pay the remaining 20 percent). Medicare Part D was added to the program in 2006 to help seniors pay for prescription drugs by enrolling in prescription insurance plans run by private companies that offer a variety of coverage choices. Part C was added to Medicare in 1997 to give Medicare beneficiaries the option to receive their Medicare benefits through private health insurance plans—called Medicare Advantage plans—instead of the government-run Parts A and B. Medicare Advantage subscribers typically pay a monthly premium to cover items not covered by Parts A and B, such as prescription drugs, dental care, vision care, and gym memberships.

to attract qualified employees. The federal government encouraged this trend by offering employers tax deductions for health care expenses and allowing the insurance benefit to be tax-free to employees. The National Labor Relations Board also ruled that health benefits could be part of collective bargaining agreements, so unions supported the employer-based system as well.

After World War II ended in 1945, employers continued to offer health insurance because it had become such a popular job benefit. As a result, this model of health insurance expanded to cover more and more workers. The benefits offered under these plans expanded as well, giving people more medical services and improvements in medical technologies. In these early postwar years, the primary insurance provider was Blue Cross. Also, because Blue Cross initially provided coverage only for hospital services, Blue Shield plans were created to cover doctor services, and the name became Blue Cross/Blue Shield. According to some estimates, more than 20 million Americans had enrolled in Blue Cross/Blue Shield plans by 1950, providing widespread coverage for many working people. Of course, the costs of the insurance rose along with improvements in care, but during the postwar period, the U.S. economy was booming and employers were happy to absorb the extra costs.

The Privatization of Health Insurance

The success of the early Blue Cross/Blue Shield plans, in turn, encouraged private commercial insurers to begin offering health insurance, and by the end of the 1950s, prominent insurance companies like Prudential, Aetna, and Metropolitan Life of New York had entered the field. The presence of these commercial companies, however, fundamentally changed the Blue Cross model of health insurance, which sought to cover everyone. According to many health care experts, the root of this transformation was that commercial insurers were not as concerned with serving the public good; as private companies, their goal was to make money. Therefore, unlike Blue Cross—which charged everyone the same premium, in effect requiring healthy people to subsidize the sick—commercial insurers sought to attract healthy people by offering them cheaper policies that more

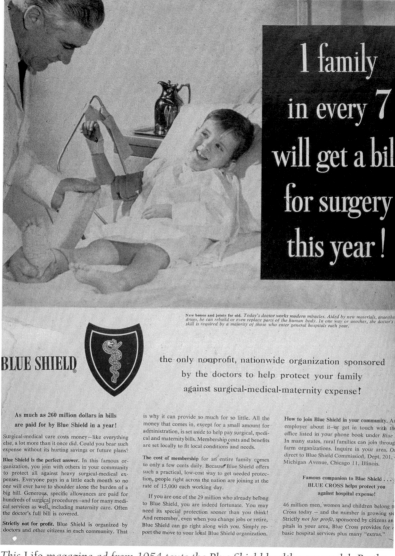

New bones and joints for old. Today's doctor works modern miracles. Aided by new materials, anaesthetic drugs, he can rebuild or even replace parts of the human body. In one way or another, the doctor's skill is required by a majority of those who enter general hospitals each year.

BLUE SHIELD

the only nonprofit, nationwide organization sponsored by the doctors to help protect your family against surgical-medical-maternity expense!

As much as 260 million dollars in bills are paid for by Blue Shield in a year!

Surgical-medical care costs money—like everything else, a lot more than it once did. Could you bear such expense without its hurting savings or future plans?

Blue Shield is the perfect answer. In this famous organization, you join with others in your community to protect all against heavy surgical-medical expenses. Everyone pays in a little each month so no one will ever have to shoulder alone the burden of a big bill. Generous, specific allowances are paid for hundreds of surgical procedures—and for many medical services as well, including maternity care. Often the doctor's full bill is covered.

Strictly not for profit. Blue Shield is organized by doctors and other citizens in each community. That

is why it can provide so much for so little. All the money that comes in, except for a small amount for administration, is set aside to help pay surgical, medical and maternity bills. Membership costs and benefits are set locally to fit local conditions and needs.

The cost of membership for an entire family comes to only a few cents daily. Because Blue Shield offers such a practical, low-cost way to get needed protection, people right across the nation are joining at the rate of 15,000 each working day.

If you are one of the 29 million who already belong to Blue Shield, you are indeed fortunate. You may need its special protection sooner than you think! And remember, even when you change jobs or retire, Blue Shield can go right along with you. Simply report the move to your local Blue Shield organization.

How to join Blue Shield in your community. As employer about it—or get in touch with the office listed in your phone book under Blue . In many states, rural families can join through farm organizations. Inquire in your area. Or direct to Blue Shield Commission, Dept. 201, Michigan Avenue, Chicago 11, Illinois.

Famous companion to Blue Shield . . . BLUE CROSS helps protect you against hospital expense!

46 million men, women and children belong to Cross today — and the number is growing ste Strictly not for profit, sponsored by citizens an pitals in your area, Blue Cross provides for basic hospital services plus many "extras."

This Life magazine ad from 1954 touts the Blue Shield health care model. By the end of the fifties commercial insurance companies had replaced the Blue Shield model with a health-care-for-profit one.

closely reflected their individual health risks. Rates were then adjusted when subscribers' health status changed. The old and those already sick, who seemed to pose the highest risk for insurers, were charged much higher rates and sometimes rejected for coverage altogether.

This strategy, known as experience rating, permitted the commercial insurers to substantially undercut the premiums offered healthy people by Blue Cross/Blue Shield. Within just a few years, enrollment in commercial insurance plans exceeded the number of people insured by Blue Cross/Blue Shield. Ultimately, the competition forced Blue Cross/Blue Shield insurers to adopt the same experience rating model used by commercial insurance firms, and the Blue Cross community rate system completely disappeared from American life. The Blue Cross model simply could not survive after the youngest, healthiest people were cherry-picked by commercial insurers. As Odin Anderson, a leading expert on health insurance, declared in 1968, "The community rate concept is, for all practical purposes, dead."[6] This death sentence was finally confirmed in 1986, when Congress officially removed the tax breaks historically provided to Blue Cross, after a finding by the U.S. Internal Revenue Service that the insurer was no longer any different from commercial insurers.

HEALTH CARE VALUE

"While it's true that we're paying 14 times as many dollars for health care as we did in 1950, we're getting an amazing return on our investment. Since 1950, the average U.S. life expectancy has increased by almost nine years."—Sally C. Pipes, president and CEO of the Pacific Research Institute, a conservative think tank that promotes free market principles.

Sally C. Pipes, *The Top Ten Myths of American Health Care: A Citizen's Guide.* San Francisco: Pacific Research Institute, 2008, p. 25.

The effect of the privatization of health insurance on the access of Americans to quality, affordable health care was dramatic. As for-profit insurers focused on insuring people in good health, sicker and older Americans found it increasingly difficult to find affordable health insurance. And as this higher-risk population was peeled away from the broader community of mostly healthy people, the costs of insuring them grew significantly. Also, since health insurance in the United States was employer-based, only people employed by large companies even stood a chance of being offered affordable health insurance coverage. The unemployed (which included large numbers of retired elderly), the self-employed, and people employed at small businesses faced the highest costs because, unlike the numerous employees of a large company, they did not have access to a large insurance pool in which risk could be spread to keep down premium costs. In fact, even when healthy individuals were willing to pay extremely high premiums, many insurers simply refused to provide policies, sometimes on controversial grounds such as race, sex, age, or occupation, which insurers defended as relevant to the amount and cost of health care the beneficiaries might use. Many health care experts therefore conclude that the privatization of health care led to higher health care costs and created a larger uninsured population in the United States. As Harvard Medical School professor Arnold S. Relman argues:

> Markets are not concerned with justice or equity. When private health care and insurance are sold in commercial markets by profit-driven providers, access is limited largely to those who can afford to pay—or those whose employers pay for them. . . . There can be little doubt that the swelling army of uninsured and underinsured, and the progressive fraying of coverage, are the result of high costs in our market-driven system.[7]

Government Health Benefits for the Poor and the Aged

Another historic change in the American health care system came in 1965, when Medicare was created to help older people deal with the rising costs of health care in the new private insurance markets. As of 1965, only about half of all seniors were covered by a health insurance plan. As a result, many seniors faced huge medical bills that they could not pay—bills that caused terrible financial hardship and were a leading cause of poverty among the elderly during this period.

U.S. president John F. Kennedy campaigned for a broad government plan to help the elderly in 1960, and after Kennedy's assassination in November 1963, the country's new president, Lyndon Baines Johnson, took up the cause of senior health care. During this period, a growing U.S. economy helped to create widespread public support for the idea of taking care of the health of older people. Congress finally acted on the issue after Johnson was elected president by a landslide in 1964, and the president signed the landmark Medicare program into law on July 30, 1965. The original Medicare program had three parts: (1) Medicare Part A, which paid for most hospital care, skilled nursing care for a limited time, and some home health care for all older Americans; (2) Medicare Part B, which paid for doctors visits as long as seniors opted for the program and paid premiums; and (3) Medicaid, a separate program, which paid for long-term nursing care for poor seniors as well as health care for other vulnerable Americans, such as the disabled and poor, single-parent families. As former senator Tom Daschle notes, "The final Medicare bill represented the largest expansion of health-care coverage in American history."[8]

With former president Harry Truman at his side President Johnson signs the Medicare bill into law on July 30, 1965.

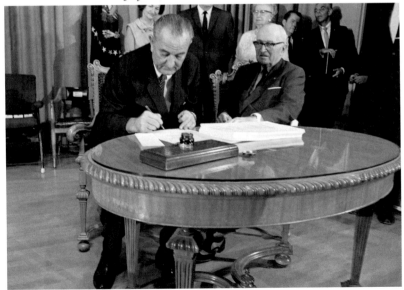

Medicare was a tremendous help to older, disabled, and very poor Americans, providing them with the health care safety net that they so desperately needed. As health care expert Marian E. Gornick explains in a 1996 article about Medicare's thirtieth anniversary, "With the implementation of Medicare on July 1, 1966, virtually the entire elderly population in the Nation was made eligible for Part A coverage, and almost all had voluntarily enrolled in Part B."[9] The out-of-pocket medical costs for these groups were significantly reduced as a direct result of the legislation. In addition, mortality rates for seniors decreased over the next few decades, and many health experts credit these declining death rates among older people, at least in part, to the increased access to medical care provided by Medicare and Medicaid.

THE HEALTH CARE INDUSTRY

"Health care is the largest industry in the United States, employing more than 14 million people nationwide. US health expenditure totaled $2.2 trillion in 2007, comprising 16.2% of the US economy."—ProCon.org, a nonprofit public charity devoted to promoting critical thinking about health care issues.

ProCon.org, "Right to Health Care," August 4, 2010. http://healthcare.procon. org/#Overview.

By removing some of the highest-risk beneficiaries from the overall pool of people needing health care and providing them with government-paid health care, the Medicare program also took the pressure off private insurers and, in this way, strengthened the private health care insurance system. However, most experts in the health field also say that Medicare helped to increase health care costs even more. In fact, as Daschle explains, "government-sponsored health insurance for the elderly turned out to be a financial windfall [for doctors, hospitals, nursing homes, and insurance companies]"[10] because it allowed them to charge higher fees than they were able to charge before Medicare.

Daschle explains, for example, that even before Medicaid began operating, Blue Cross and hospital groups convinced federal officials to pay hospitals and nursing homes not only for expenses but also a 2 percent bonus, which Medicare pays without investigating whether the fees are too high. Instead, hospitals and nursing homes were permitted to pick "fiscal intermediaries" to make this determination, and most of the intermediaries tended to be insurance companies, who were then paid for their administrative costs. Later, for-profit nursing homes, for-profit hospitals, and nonprofit nursing homes were granted a reimbursement formula that pays them for allowable cost plus a 7.5 percent profit—a formula known as cost-plus. Doctors also benefited because they charged as much as they could to the government with little oversight. The result, many health care experts agree, was a rapid rise in the cost of health care, which continued in later decades. According to Relman, "The average rate of increase in health expenditures since the late 1960s has been between 9 and 10 percent per year, which is more than twice the rate of general price inflation."[11]

Rising Costs and Managed Care

The soaring health care costs in the 1960s, 1970s, and 1980s led to efforts to control costs through managed care—a term that generally refers to health insurance plans that seek to exercise control over the quantity and quality of health care services provided to beneficiaries, rather than simply pay the bills submitted by medical providers. Employers were at the forefront of the push for managed care because they had experienced decades of unpredictable and uncontrolled premium increases for their employees, only part of which employers could ask employees to pay. The managed care plans typically offered much cheaper premium rates to employers and beneficiaries than typical health insurance plans.

One of the first types of low-cost managed care plans was developed in the early 1970s and was called the health maintenance organization (HMO). The first HMOs, like the early Blue Cross plans, were nonprofits that sought to emphasize preventive care and provide health care at a lower cost by restricting beneficiaries to a network of medical providers who agreed to various rules geared toward reducing costs. As insurance expert Corinne Mitchell explains,

> When HMO Plans were first introduced, members paid a fixed, prepaid monthly premium in exchange for health care from a contracted network of providers. The contracted network of providers includes hospitals, clinics and health care providers that have signed a contract with the HMO. In this sense, HMOs are the most restrictive form of managed care plans because they restrict the procedures, providers and benefits by requiring that the members use these providers and no others.[12]

The federal government also subsidized HMOs, helping them to proliferate. In 1973, President Richard Nixon signed the Health Maintenance Organization Act—a law that allocated millions in grants and loans to HMOs and provided incentives for employers to offer them as an option along with traditional health insurance

Dr. Paul Elwood authored the health plan called the health maintenance organization in 1970 and saw his ideas incorporated in the Health Maintenance Organization Act signed by President Nixon in 1973.

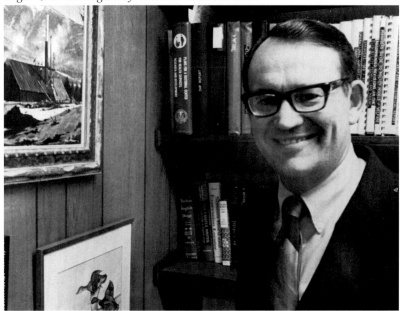

National Health Expenditures and Their Share of Gross Domestic Product, 1960–2008

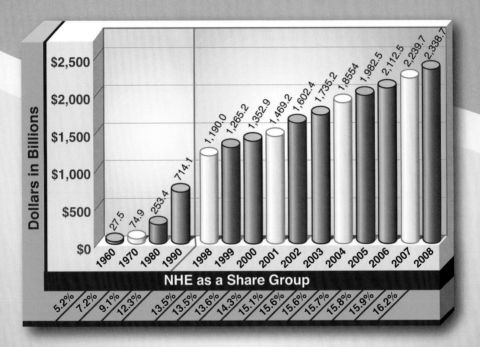

Dollars in Billions

1960	27.5
1970	74.9
1980	253.4
1990	714.1
1998	1,190.0
1999	1,265.2
2000	1,352.9
2001	1,469.2
2002	1,602.4
2003	1,735.2
2004	1,855.4
2005	1,982.5
2006	2,112.5
2007	2,239.7
2008	2,338.7

NHE as a Share Group

5.2% 7.2% 9.1% 12.3% 13.5% 13.5% 13.6% 14.3% 15.1% 15.6% 15.6% 15.7% 15.8% 15.9% 16.2%

Taken from: Centers for Medicare and Medicaid Services, Office of the Actuary, National Health Statistics Group. At http://www.cms.hhs.gov/NationalHealthExpendData.

plans. By the mid-1990s, more insured Americans were enrolled in managed care plans than in traditional health care plans.

The HMO plans were successful for a while at holding down health care costs, but over time most HMOs became more and more restrictive. They frequently imposed onerous conditions on doctors such as requiring them to see more patients and obtain preapproval before providing many types of medical services. The HMOs also began to deny many claims for medical care submitted by beneficiaries, claiming they were too expensive or unnecessary. Commentators say that these actions were taken by HMOs largely because many insurers in the HMO industry made bad investments in real estate deals. When the real estate market crashed during the savings and loan crisis in the 1980s, many HMOs were unable to cover all their claims. Whatever the original reason behind the HMO transformation,

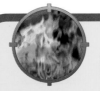

Free Medical Clinics in America

With close to 47 million Americans uninsured and the U.S. economy in a recession, the only places many people in the United States can turn to for medical care are free medical clinics organized by private groups funded mostly by states or private donations. Many of these groups started out as private charities to provide medical care to the poor in underdeveloped countries, but in recent years, the need for the free medical services in the United States is growing so rapidly that the clinics cannot keep up with demand. The National Association of Free Clinics (NAFC), an organization dedicated to supporting the free clinics, estimates, for example, that free clinics saw 4 million patients in 2008, but that figure doubled to 8 million in 2009. According to estimates by some clinic organizers, roughly 83 percent of patients seen in the clinics come from working households, often homes where parents are working two or three part-time jobs, but usually these are jobs that do not provide health insurance. Some free clinics have permanent locations, while others are organized as health fairs where doctors, dentists, and other medical providers donate their time to see as many patients as possible in a clinic that might last a few days. When one of these temporary clinics is scheduled to come to an area, people often camp out overnight to be first in line so that they can be seen. Dental care is one of the most pressing needs, because even if people are covered by insurance or Medicaid, dentistry often is not a covered service. Even if health care reform is effective in covering more people with health insurance, therefore, free clinic organizers predict a great and continuing need for free medical services, even in the world's richest nation.

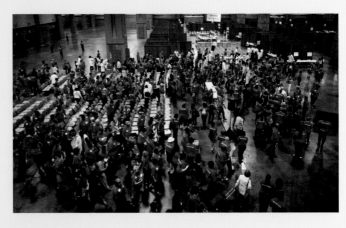

Volunteers ready to open a massive free clinic sponsored by the National Association of Free Clinics in Washington, D.C., in August 2010.

however, the industry continued to maintain this new restrictive approach even after its financial condition improved. Some commentators suggest the reason is that the HMO industry, like the early traditional health insurers, had become by this time a for-profit endeavor that saw profits in the new restrictions. As a result, however, HMOs have become much less popular than they once were, as well as less affordable.

As HMOs declined, insurers began to promote another form of managed care—preferred provider organization (PPO) insurance. Under PPO plans, subscribers select physicians from a group of doctors who have agreed to be preferred providers for that insurance company, but patients are still free to consult specialists (from a list of preferred providers) without a referral from their primary doctor. Theoretically, insurance companies can control costs through these plans by getting preferred providers to agree to negotiated fee schedules. However, largely because patients have unimpeded access to specialists, the cost of medical care under PPOs has become more expensive than under the HMO model.

A National Health Care Crisis

Health care costs continued to skyrocket in the late 1990s and early 2000s, pressuring employers and causing many, especially smaller, companies to reduce or completely eliminate health care benefits for employees. Other employers are struggling to maintain health insurance but are changing to policies that have higher deductibles or that require employees to shoulder more of the cost. Premiums for individual health insurance policies have also risen greatly, making health insurance often completely unaffordable for many self-employed or unemployed individuals, as well as for the ever-growing number of working people not covered by an employer policy. And people who are sick or have preexisting conditions—broadly interpreted by health insurance companies to mean any evidence of a health problem prior to signing up for a health insurance policy—often find it impossible to find coverage at any cost. Because so many Americans are now underinsured or without coverage, most health experts agree that America is once again facing a health care crisis—a crisis that has prompted repeated attempts at reform and spurred a national health care debate.

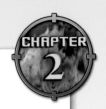
THE DEBATE ABOUT HEALTH CARE REFORM

As the costs of health care rose throughout the twentieth century, a number of attempts were made to reform the health care system in order to provide affordable and effective health care for all Americans. In fact, presidents from Franklin Delano Roosevelt to the present day have pushed for various types of health care reform, but many of these failed due to opposition from the American Medical Association (AMA) and the health insurance industry, which time after time successfully portrayed reforms as "socialized medicine." Today, as health care costs continue their meteoric rise and increasing numbers of Americans find themselves without access to affordable health care, the historic debate about health care reform continues. This policy and political debate is as contentious as ever, revealing vastly differing views about some of the thorniest health care issues, such as how to preserve quality care, how to provide health care for everyone, and how to control health care costs.

A History of Reform Efforts

One of the very first health care reform efforts was made by the American Association of Labor Legislation (AALL)—an organization of progressive reformers active during the early part of the twentieth century. The group's 1915 model health care bill proposed comprehensive national health insurance coverage for the working class and the poor, with program costs shared among workers (40 percent), employers (20 percent), and the state (20 percent). At first, the AALL proposal seemed destined to succeed, but it eventually failed due to opposition from three highly influential groups—the American Medical Association (AMA), the American Federation of Labor, and commercial insurers. As public health expert Karen S. Palmer explains, "Opposition from doctors, labor, insurance companies, and business contributed to the failure of Progressives to achieve compulsory national health insurance."[13] The U.S. entry into World War I against Germany in 1917 sealed the fate of the AALL bill, as anti-German sentiment grew in America and opponents of health reform associated it with German socialism—a political ideology in which the government controls most or all of the nation's economy.

The idea of national health insurance arose again in the 1930s, after America sank into the Great Depression—a worldwide economic slowdown in which millions of Americans lost their jobs, their homes, and their fortunes. Faced with this unprecedented challenge, Roosevelt created a Committee on Economic Security to study the problems of economic insecurity and offer solutions as part of his New Deal legislative platform. The

When Franklin Roosevelt signed the Social Security Act in 1935, it included old age pensions and unemployment insurance but no health care provisions, though they were originally planned.

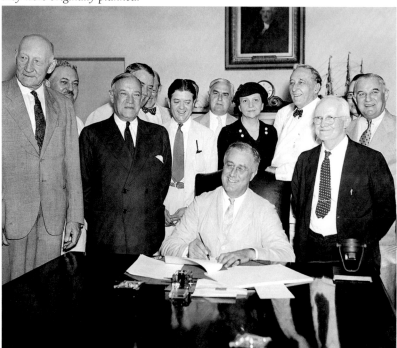

Committee studied four types of social insurance—unemployment insurance, public employment and relief, old age security, and medical care—and it included a national health care plan in its report to the president. However, in the face of AMA opposition that was based on doctors' fears that they would lose money or their autonomy, Roosevelt decided not to push for health insurance to be part of the legislative social security bill that was working its way through Congress, for fear that it would ruin his chances to get other important programs enacted. As a result, Roosevelt's 1935 Social Security Act—which set up a broad program of old age, disability, and unemployment insurance—did not include any type of national health insurance. Because of the Depression, unemployment and old age benefits simply ranked higher in the president's list of national priorities.

A History of Reform Attempts

"America has been working on providing access to health care for all Americans since the nineteen-thirties, the nineteen-forties, the nineteen-fifties, the nineteen-sixties, nineteen-seventies, nineteen-eighties, and the nineteen-nineties."—Sheila Jackson-Lee, a Democratic congresswoman from Texas.

Quoted in Jill Lepore, "Preexisting Condition," *New Yorker*, December 7, 2009. www.newyorker.com/talk/comment/2009/12/07/091207taco_talk_lepore.

A later proposal for national health care introduced into the Congress by New York senator Robert F. Wagner met the same fate, and Roosevelt died in April 1945 without offering another health insurance proposal. As Palmer explains, "Just as the AALL campaign ran into the declining forces of progressivism and then WWI, the movement for national health insurance in the 1930's ran into the declining fortunes of the New Deal and then WWII."[14]

When World War II ended in 1945, the next U.S. president, Harry Truman, also came out strongly in favor of a universal, comprehensive national health insurance plan. However, Truman's reform efforts ultimately succumbed, like earlier reforms, to strong opposition from the AMA and its allies, who called Truman's bill "socialized medicine" because it would involve too much government control. Anti-Communist sentiment was rampant throughout this Cold War era—the period following WWII when the United States and Russia maintained an openly hostile relationship due to differing political ideologies—and Russian communism, like socialism, was an ideology in which the government exerts control over most or all facets of the economy.

In fact, the first major U.S. health care reform did not happen until twenty years later, when Johnson created Medicare/Medicaid in 1965. This milestone law finally achieved some of the health care goals sought by Roosevelt and Truman. The signing ceremony for the new law was even held in Independence, Missouri, the home of ex-president Truman, so that he could attend. However, Medicare only provided health care insurance for the old, the disabled, and the poor; many working and middle-class families who did not have health insurance through employers were still left without affordable health insurance.

The first modern push for reform that would provide universal health insurance for all Americans occurred in 1971 when various candidates were campaigning to be their party's presidential candidate in the 1972 presidential election. Republican president Richard Nixon supported a market-based approach that continued America's employer-based system of health insurance, while Democratic senator Edward Kennedy supported a government-run program, similar to Medicare. After Nixon was reelected president, he introduced his Comprehensive Health Insurance Act—a bill that required employers to purchase health insurance for employees but also set up a federal health plan available to Americans on a sliding scale based on income. This legislation, however, ultimately became the victim of Watergate—a political scandal that undermined support for Nixon and his programs.

Despite rising health care costs, neither of the next two presidents—Republican Gerald Ford nor Democrat Jimmy Carter—was able to make headway on health care reforms. Ironically, President Ronald Reagan, a conservative Republican elected in 1980 who once called Medicare the first step on the road to socialism, helped to enact the 1988 Medicare Catastrophic Coverage Act (MCCA)—the biggest expansion of Medicare since its creation in 1965. The original Medicare program only paid for hospital stays of up to ninety days, but the MCCA provided seniors with full hospital coverage (after certain deductibles). In addition, the act provided a host of other new benefits, such as prescription drug costs and extended skilled nursing and home health care. Reagan's bill paid for these new costs by charging wealthier Medicare recipients a surtax of up to eight hundred dollars per year. Yet this victory for seniors proved to be short-lived, because the new tax on affluent seniors caused such a groundswell of opposition that Congress decided to repeal the law just a year later, in 1989.

Following the MCCA fiasco, it was not until President Bill Clinton took office in 1993 that health care reform once again became part of the national agenda. Clinton set up a task force on the issue headed by then First Lady Hillary Clinton. The Clinton proposal, called the Health Security Act, required that all Americans be covered by health insurance either through

In 1993 Hillary Clinton met with seniors as part of the information campaign for the Clintons' proposed Health Security Act.

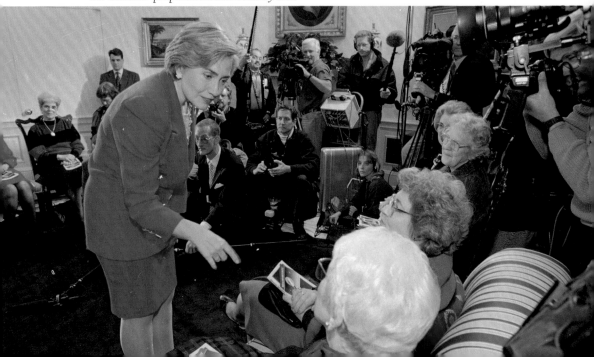

their employers or through government-run regional alliances, with competition among insurers regulated by the government. However, like other attempts to create universal health insurance, the bill was attacked for allowing too much government control over health care. Ultimately, the Clinton bill was defeated by a media campaign mounted by insurance industry lobbyists. The campaign was called "Harry and Louise" and featured ordinary Americans criticizing the bill as too complex and bureaucratic. The defeat of the Clinton health care reform package largely pushed the issue to the political sidelines until the 2008 presidential election.

The Best Health Care in the World or a Broken System?

The political debate about how to solve the health care crisis continues to be highly polarized, with few areas of agreement. Views differ even on the most basic question of whether health care reform is needed. Many Republicans and other conservatives insist, for example, that the current free market system of health care and health care insurance in the United States provides the best health care in the world. As Republican president George W. Bush said in a 2004 presidential debate, "Our healthcare system is the envy of the world."[15] Conservatives point out that people from other nations often come to the United States for medical care because America offers such cutting-edge treatments and technologies. Karl Rove, former deputy chief of staff to Bush, notes some of these accomplishments: "From 1998 to 2002 nearly twice as many new drugs were launched in the U.S. as in Europe. According to the U.S. Pharmaceutical Industry Report, some 2,900 new drugs are now being researched here. America's five top hospitals conduct more clinical trials than all the hospitals in any other developed country."[16]

As a result, many on the political right argue that the existing system of private health insurance and medical care is not broken and should not be fundamentally changed. As Rove states, "[The] trashing of American health care as 'a broken system' . . . doesn't resonate with most Americans. They are happy about their health care, doctor and hospital. [A 2009] . . . poll found that 83%

A Health Care Tragedy

As the country was debating health care reform legislation, the Democratic National Committee created a website to collect stories from people around the country about their experiences. Here is one of those stories, submitted by Kathy from Texas:

Jessica Leanne Hurt died on June 13, 2009. She was 21 years old. Jessica had gallstones, which could have been fixed by a fairly minor surgical procedure. Although there is a crisis in this country, with over 45 million people uninsured, that was not Jessica's situation. She was employed and had health insurance.

As the gallstone problem developed she sought treatment and surgery was recommended. However, she was informed that she would be required to pay $5000 upfront to cover her deductible and co-pay before she could have surgery. She tried several hospitals, in an attempt to work out a payment plan, but was unable to find one willing to work with her. As her pain increased she ended up in the emergency room on several occasions, but each time she was sent home with nothing but pain medication. She grew sicker over the next few months and working became increasingly difficult. Eventually she lost her job, and with it her insurance, because she missed work too often. On the evening of May 22nd, in tremendous pain, she went to the emergency room again. This time she was sick enough that the hospital admitted her, even without insurance. By morning she was in ICU [intensive care unit] with pancreatitis and sepsis. Her kidneys had failed and her liver was starting to also. Her body was shutting down. The doctors and nurses worked desperately to save her as her family and friends waited and prayed. She was on a ventilator and dialysis, in and out of consciousness, for three weeks before she died. During the time that she was in the ICU, now unemployed, uninsured, and gravely disabled, Jessica qualified for Medicaid; thankfully, because her hospital bill rose to over $400,000. In an extraordinary example of the system being penny wise and dollar foolish, Jessica Hurt died and almost half a million taxpayer dollars were spent because a $5000 upfront payment was required. I don't know what the answer is, but our system is broken and something needs to change."

Kathy from Port Arthur, TX, "Health Care Stories for America," Health Care Action Center, 2010. http://stories.barackobama.com/healthcare/stories/189574.

of Americans are very or somewhat satisfied with the quality of care they and their families receive."[17] In fact, even though many employers are opting to scale back or eliminate health insurance coverage for workers, the U.S. Census Bureau estimates that as of 2008, 58.5 percent of Americans still benefit from having their insurance premiums paid, at least in part, by their employers. Republicans have a point, therefore, when they say that a significant segment of voters would simply prefer to keep their current insurance and are lukewarm about any type of health care reform.

NO UNIVERSAL CARE

"Despite all the rights and privileges and entitlements that Americans enjoy today, we have never decided to provide medical care for everybody who needs it."—T.R. Reid, a longtime correspondent for the *Washington Post* and a commentator for National Public Radio.

T.R. Reid, *The Healing of America: The Global Quest for Better, Cheaper, and Fairer Health Care*. New York: Penguin, 2009, p. 2.

Most Democrats and political progressives, on the other hand, maintain that the American health care system only provides good health care for the rich, leaving increasingly large portions of the population without access to affordable health care or health insurance. They cite a 1986 report by the Institute of Medicine (IOM), for example, which found significant deficiencies and variations in the quality of U.S. medical care. Similarly, a review of the world's health care systems in 2000 by the World Health Organization (WHO), a United Nations health agency, ranked the United States behind nearly every other industrialized country in terms of the quality of its medical care, most especially in promoting equitable care. As Daschle argues: "At the dawn of the twenty-first century, we are the only industrialized nation that does not guarantee necessary health care to all of its citizens. It is stunning and shameful."[18]

According to a 2009 IOM report, these uninsured Americans tend to forgo health care and are more likely to suffer from un-

necessary illness, greater limitations in quality of life, and pre-
mature death. In fact, the IOM estimates that the lack of health
insurance leads to eighteen thousand unnecessary deaths each
year. Not having health insurance can also quickly bankrupt a
family in the event of a medical emergency. Even people who are
insured find that their insurance pays only around 80 percent of
major medical bills, so the insured are at risk, too, in the event of
serious illness or injury. According to a recent study published in
the *American Journal of Medicine*, "Using a conservative definition,
62.1% of all bankruptcies in 2007 were medical. . . . Most medical debtors were well educated, owned homes, and had middle-
class occupations. Three quarters had health insurance."[19] This
situation, many experts believe, frays the fabric of civil society as
well as the economy, weakening America from the inside.

*Approximately 62 percent of 2007 bankruptcies were medical, and most medical
debtors were well educated, homeowners, had middle-class occupations, and had
health insurance.*

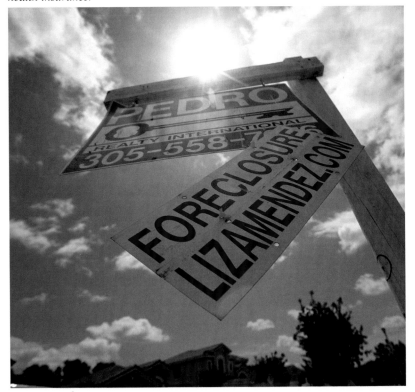

The Role of Government—Competing Visions

Among those policy makers who agree that the U.S. health care system needs improvement, perhaps the biggest disagreement is over the role of government. The majority of conservatives favor keeping today's private market system in which not only the medical providers but also health insurers are for-profit entities. Reforming this system, according to conservative analysts, hinges on empowering patients to be intelligent consumers of health care services so that they can choose their medical services and insurance and pay a larger share of health care costs. As Republican George P. Shultz, former U.S. secretary of state, explains, "The first step [in health care reform] is to ensure that consumers have a significant financial stake in the system and an ability to make informed decisions about their own health care coverage."[20]

UNSUSTAINABLE COSTS

"[U.S. health care] costs, many of which are unnecessary, are on the road to levels that cannot be sustained."—George P. Shultz, a former U.S. secretary of state during the Ronald Reagan administration and currently a fellow at the conservative think tank the Hoover Institution.

George P. Shultz and John B. Shoven, *Putting Our House in Order: A Guide to Social Security and Health Care Reform.* New York: W.W. Norton, 2008, p. 137.

Conservatives would create this financial stake by requiring people to purchase individual health insurance plans with high deductibles, so that they have to pay for all medical costs below the deductible. Another way of encouraging consumer-driven health care is the health savings account (HSA)—a medical savings account that currently allows people to set aside up to $2,700 ($5,450 for families) each year to pay for medical expenses, tax-exempt. The basic idea is that if patients have more of a stake in health care they will demand higher quality of care, and the competition for these health consumers will lower health care costs. Conservatives point to certain types of health care that are already competitive because they are typically not covered by insurance—such as laser eye surgery—and note that free market competition in these services has led both to quality improvements and to falling prices.

Liberals and progressives, however, disagree with the consumer model; they are convinced that the private market will not save the U.S. health care system. Asking people to pay more for health care when they already cannot afford basic care, they say, would only leave more people outside the system. And a consumer model, opponents say, would put patients in the position of deciding what care they need instead of their doctors. As Relman argues,

> The important tasks of evaluating and interpreting symptoms, of coordinating and integrating services for each patient, and of deciding which specialty services and which institutions and facilities would best meet the needs of each patient would be left to the patients themselves. Most patients would be daunted by such responsibility and few could take it on.[21]

Instead, many progressives favor a government-run health care system. They envision a single-payer government insurance plan financed by taxes—a plan similar to Medicare in which all Americans would be covered for basic health care by a government insurance fund, with private doctors and hospitals paid by this fund. During recent debates, this basic idea has been called by various names—Medicare for all, single-payer, or the public option. The advantages of such a program, proponents say, are many: Only one public insurance agency would be accountable to voters; no or few co-pays, deductibles, or yearly or lifetime limits; no sales and marketing or profit concerns; small administrative costs; and low, negotiated prices for drugs, medical services, and medical equipment. According to many progressives, this type of public health care system eliminates the private sector profit motive from health care—the central problem in the current system and the key reason for denials of care. As Cynthia Tucker, editorial page editor for the *Atlanta Journal-Constitution*, explains, "The for-profit health insurance industry is in the business of maximizing profits for their shareholders, and the only way they can do that is to hold down the payments they make for medical care."[22]

Proposals for government-run health plans, however, have always run into a wall of opposition from conservatives, who often equate them with socialism and raise fears about government bureaucracy and a loss of freedom to choose medical providers. Supporters of the public option dismiss these criticisms, pointing out that truly Socialist health care means that the government would own all the hospitals and directly employ doctors and other providers—a system far different from Medicare, in which providers are privately owned and chosen by patients. Of course, a Medicare-for-all system would take business away from commercial insurance companies—a result that helps explain the industry's historical opposition to government-run reform proposals.

Providing Universal Health Care

A major goal of most health reform proposals, however, is universal care—making it available to everyone who needs it, not just those who are healthy or who can afford it. To many health care experts, basic health care is a human right that all people should have, especially citizens of the United States, one of the wealthiest countries in the world. Others disagree, noting that the right to other basic needs is also not God-given nor constitutional. They say health care, like food, shelter, or clothing, is just another type of commodity in the private marketplace. Yet it is true that many nations, including the United States, provide a government safety net for the poor to provide for basic needs, and Medicare basically added health care to this list, at least for older Americans. Progressives argue that a civilized society like America's should offer health care for all Americans as part of this safety net.

Part of the problem of extending health care to everyone, however, is that younger, healthier people have less need for health care and may not want to pay for it, either directly or through taxes. Yet just as the original Blue Cross programs were based on the idea of spreading the risk, a system of universal

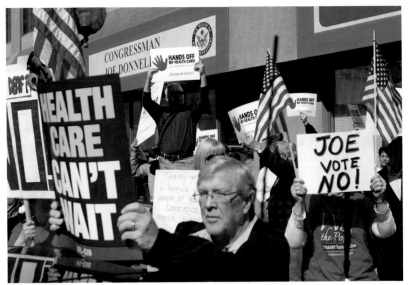

The health care debate is divided along political lines with Republicans favoring no government involvement in health care and the Democrats for it.

health care is not possible unless a broad pool of people is insured, so that the young and healthy help subsidize the sick and, in turn, are covered when they might need medical care. Many health reform proposals, therefore, have included provisions that compel individuals or employers to either provide health insurance or pay a penalty. Like other parts of reform, however, this compulsory health insurance concept has been controversial, both with small employers, who say they cannot afford it, and with conservatives, who see it as another government infringement on basic individual freedoms.

Controlling Health Care Costs

Perhaps the most difficult challenge in reforming health care is controlling costs, which surpassed $2.3 trillion in 2008, over eight times the amount spent in 1980. Almost everyone agrees that costs have reached unsustainable levels, but there is significant disagreement about both the cause of rising costs and the appropriate solutions. According to the independent health care think tank the Kaiser Family Foundation, the major drivers of health care costs are new medical technologies and prescription

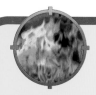

A Health Care Industry Whistle-Blower

Wendell Potter, a former director of corporate communications for the health insurance company Cigna, is an insurance company insider who became a whistle-blower who claims that the insurance industry is solely interested in profits. Potter retired from Cigna in May 2008 after he became disillusioned with the industry's efforts to shift health costs to individuals. In June 2009, Potter testified before a congressional committee about insurance company practices, explaining:

> The top priority of for-profit companies is to drive up the value of their stock. . . . [F]or-profit insurers must prove that they made more money during the previous quarter than a year earlier and that the portion of the premium going to medical costs is falling. . . . To help meet Wall Street's relentless profit expectations, insurers routinely dump policyholders who are less profitable or who get sick. Insurers have several ways to cull the sick from their rolls. One is policy rescission. They look carefully to see if a sick policyholder may have omitted a minor illness, a pre-existing condition, when applying for coverage, and then they use that as justification to cancel the policy, even if the enrollee has never missed a premium payment. . . . They also dump small businesses whose employees' medical claims exceed what insurance underwriters expected. All it takes is one illness or accident among employees at a small business to prompt an insurance company to hike the next year's premiums so high that the employer has to cut benefits, shop for another carrier, or stop offering coverage altogether—leaving workers uninsured. The practice is known in the industry as "purging."

> What we have today . . . is a Wall Street–run system that has proven itself an untrustworthy partner to its customers, to the doctors and hospitals who deliver care, and to the state and federal governments that attempt to regulate it.

Wendell Potter, "Testimony of Wendell Potter, Philadelphia, PA, before the U.S. Senate Committee on Commerce, Science and Transportation," June 24, 2009. www.pbs.org/moyers/journal/07102009/potter_testimony.html.

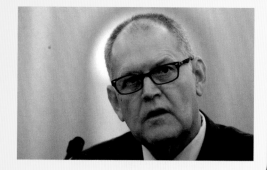

Former CIGNA spokesman Wendell Potter testified before Congress about insurance companies practice of "purging" people off of health insurance.

drugs, chronic disease, the aging of the U.S. population, and high administrative costs.

Many health experts on the political left argue that the government-run Medicare model is more efficient than the private insurance system, pointing out that private insurers have much higher administrative costs. There is support for this argument; according to Kaiser, for example, "It is estimated that at least 7% of health care expenditures are for [insurers'] administrative costs (e.g., marketing, billing) [but] . . . this portion is much lower in the Medicare program (<2%)."[23] In fact, progressives often argue that the privatization of health care and health insurance is the real root of rising costs. As Relman explains, "The incentives in [a private health care] . . . system reward and stimulate the delivery of more services. That is why medical expenditures in the U.S. are so much higher than in any other country, and are rising more rapidly."[24]

HIGH HEALTH INSURANCE PREMIUMS

"The average American family's premiums now exceed the gross annual income of a full-time minimum wage worker." —Andrew Weil, a graduate of Harvard Medical School and founder and director of the Arizona Center for Integrative Medicine at the University of Arizona, where he is a professor of medicine and public health.

Andrew Weil, *Why Our Health Matters: A Vision of Medicine That Can Transform Our Future.* New York: Hudson Street, 2009, p. 7.

Conservatives, on the other hand, contend that the main problem is that patients do not directly pay for health care costs because medical bills are paid either by insurers or the government, causing overuse of medical services. As economist Stan Lebowitz argues in an analysis for the libertarian Cato Institute, "Overuse is the rational response of consumers who do not have to pay the entire cost of the medical services they use. The causes of those excess costs are Medicaid, Medicare, and tax laws that provide incentives for individuals to have their employers purchase their medical care in the form of private health insurance."[25] Conservatives point to a Rand study from the 1970s, which found that patients who paid larger co-payments for health care tended to use fewer medical services. Another contributor to high costs, according to conservatives, is fear of malpractice suits, which they say causes doctors and hospitals to order unnecessary tests and procedures to avoid being sued.

Consequently, progressives favor cost solutions aimed at reducing the profit motive through more government regulation of health care, while conservatives emphasize solutions geared toward increasing consumer involvement in health care (as well as making it harder to file malpractice claims). An array of other more neutral solutions has also been proposed, including: converting to electronic medical records; improving quality and efficiency in various ways; changing payment systems to reward providers for outcomes rather than each medical service; and emphasizing preventive health care services. However, the lack of consensus on cost solutions is a key reason that health care reform has been so difficult for America for so long.

HEALTH CARE SYSTEMS IN OTHER COUNTRIES

As the United States struggled with its health care policies throughout the twentieth century, other developed countries around the world faced similar health care challenges. Most other developed nations, however, chose to adopt national health insurance programs that provide near-universal coverage. In the early to mid-1900s, for example, various European countries enacted government-run health insurance programs to cover all or most citizens, albeit with a number of variations on how this is accomplished. Yet in the United States, policy makers strongly resisted the idea of a nationwide program for health care, preferring instead to give the private market almost free rein in this sector. The result, as the Institute of Medicine (IOM) explains, is: "Although America leads the world in spending on health care, it is the only wealthy, industrialized nation that does not ensure that all citizens have coverage."[26]

The European Example

In Europe, the push for health insurance began even before the United States began addressing the issue—in the late 1800s and early 1900s. Most European countries began by enacting government-run sickness insurance, to pay workers for time lost from work when they were sick. Germany developed one of the first sick pay systems in 1883, but many other countries followed, including Austria, Hungary, Norway, Britain, Russia, and the Netherlands. Other European countries, such as Sweden, Denmark, France, and Switzerland, chose instead to subsidize worker groups that provided a similar benefit. Programs did not cover all workers at first, and they did not pay for

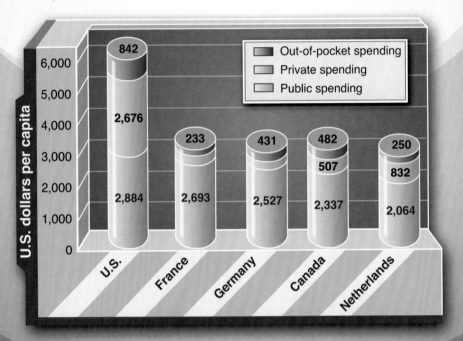

Is European Health Care More Cost-Effective?

Research consistently indicates lower overall spending on health care by European nations compared with combined U.S. public and private health care expenditures.

U.S. dollars per capita

Legend:
- Out-of-pocket spending
- Private spending
- Public spending

U.S.: 842, 2,676, 2,884
France: 233, 2,693
Germany: 431, 2,527
Canada: 482, 507, 2,337
Netherlands: 250, 832, 2,064

Taken from: Organization for Economic Cooperation and Development Health Data, 2007.

medical services initially, but they were the beginnings of universal health insurance in Europe. Later, each European country developed its own national health care system, covering all or most citizens but reflecting each country's individual history, politics, economics, and values. As Palmer notes, "Other developed countries have had some form of social insurance (that later evolved into national insurance) for nearly as long as the US has been trying to get it."[27]

According to journalist and health care writer T.R. Reid, health care systems in Europe and the world's other developed countries tend to follow one of three general models. The first model, the Bismarck (named after German chancellor Otto von Bismarck), is found in Germany, France, Belgium, and Switzerland, and has been adopted by Japan and countries in Latin America. It is the closest to the current U.S. system. In this system, like America's system, health care providers and insurers are private entities, and the program is financed by employers and employees. However, unlike the U.S. system, insurers are required by the government to cover everyone, insurers are not permitted to make a profit, and costs are controlled by tight government regulation of medical services and fees.

The health care system used in Britain, Italy, Spain, and most of Scandinavia, according to Reid, is a very different type of model called the Beverage (named after William Beverage, a British social reformer). In this type of system, the government both provides and pays for all health care, financing it with taxes. Doctors are paid by the government, and clinics and hospitals are government-owned. Medical treatment is a public benefit for everyone, and no one pays out of pocket for any health care.

SOCIALIZED MEDICINE

"Contrary to conventional American wisdom, most developed countries manage health care without resorting to 'socialized medicine.'"—T.R. Reid, a longtime correspondent for the *Washington Post* and a commentator for National Public Radio.

T.R. Reid, *The Healing of America: The Global Quest for Better, Cheaper, and Fairer Health Care*. New York: Penguin, 2009, p. 3.

The third type of health care system in the developed world is the national health insurance model—a combination of the Bismarck and the Beverage models, in which medical providers are private but the government runs the system and pays the bills. This system is similar to the U.S. Medicare program and is used in Canada, Taiwan, and South Korea.

The rest of the world—that is, most developing nations— is generally too poor to have developed any type of organized health care. Reid calls this model the out-of-pocket system, because people must pay for all medical services out of pocket. As

Reid says, "The basic rule in such countries is simple, and brutal: The rich get medical care; the poor stay sick or die."[28]

Germany's Public/Private Mix

A more detailed review of several foreign health care systems illustrates how each of these models works. In Germany, which follows the Bismarck model, most employees are required by the government to select one of more than two hundred private, non-profit insurance companies called sickness funds. These funds are required by the government to cover everyone who applies; they are not permitted to deny insurance based on preexisting conditions. The funds negotiate prices with doctors and hospitals on a regional basis, and the negotiated prices then become the fixed medical price that must be charged. As in America, doctors and hospitals are private and are permitted to make a profit. Health care in Germany, however, is not financed by taxes as is the U.S. Medicare system; instead, patients pay a monthly premium to an insurance company, and employers pay the rest. Significantly, the amount each German employee pays for health insurance is based on his or her income—a feature important in German culture. As National Public Radio correspondent Richard Knox explains: "Basing premiums on a percentage-of-salary means that the less people make, the less they have to pay. The more money they make, the more they pay. This principle is at the heart of the system. Germans call it 'solidarity.' The idea is that everybody's in it together, and nobody should be without health insurance."[29] Germany also has a private health care system which is used by the self-employed, civil servants, and anyone earning more than $72,000 per year who chooses to opt out of the public health care system. Most people do not opt out, but those who do pay private, for-profit insurance companies a premium for benefit packages, as many Americans do. The difference between the U.S. and German insurers, however, is that German insurance companies are very heavily regulated by the government, so insurers cannot raise rates after subscribers get sick or as they get older.

According to most assessments, German health benefits are very generous: no deductibles, and all Germans get the same coverage. Moreover, health insurance is continuous so that Germans

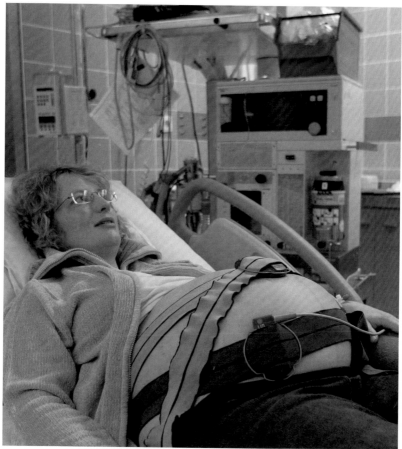

In Germany the amount a person pays for health insurance is based on income.

do not lose coverage when they lose their jobs; instead, government unemployment benefits pay for coverage until workers find new jobs, no matter how long it takes. Because of rising health care costs in recent years, adults may have to pay very small deductibles each quarter to see their doctors or pick up prescriptions, but virtually all care for children is covered until they are eighteen years old, even dental services such as orthodontia. Patients also usually do not have to wait long to get surgery or tests, and people can call a central phone number after hours and be connected to a doctor. And German sickness funds compete to provide the best benefits, offering options such as health spas, alternative therapies, and home assistance—such as cooking, cleaning, childcare, or nursing care—when patients return home after a major operation or after childbirth. As German economist Karl Lauterbach explains, German insurers compete even though they are nonprofits "because the executives earn more money, and higher prestige, if they have a larger pool of insured members."[30] This basic system has worked in Germany for more than a century.

Great Britain's National Health Service

The British health care system, a Beverage model system enacted in 1948, is an example of truly socialized medicine. Under the country's national health program, called the National Health Service (NHS), health care is provided to all by the national government and is funded by taxpayers, with no private insurers involved. The government owns the hospitals, pays the doctors, and buys all prescriptions. The central idea behind this system is that the government should provide comprehensive medical

The National Health Service in Great Britain is considered by most health care experts to be the most cost-efficient health care system in the world.

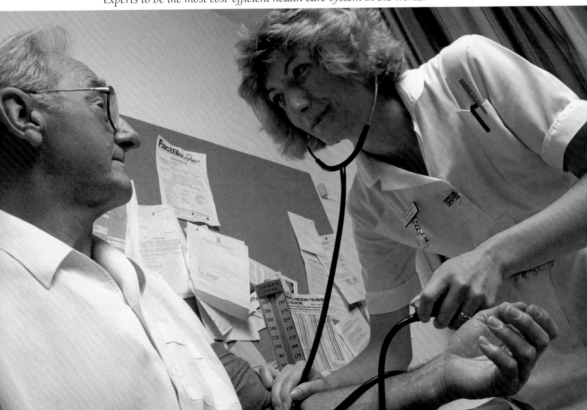

care for everyone as a fundamental social service with no fee at the point of service. As Reid describes it, "The British National Health Service . . . is dedicated to the proposition that nobody should ever have to pay a medical bill. In the NHS, there is no insurance premium to pay, no co-payment, no fee at all, whether you drop by the GP's [general practitioner's] office with a cold or receive a quadruple bypass from the nation's top cardiac surgeon."[31] This British system has been compared with the health care that America provides for its military personnel and veterans through the U.S. Department of Veterans Affairs. Most British people have grown up with this system and consider it an indispensable part of British life.

NOT THE BEST HEALTH CARE IN THE WORLD

"The World Health Organization recently rated America thirty-seventh in health outcomes, on a par with Serbia."—Andrew Weil, a graduate of Harvard Medical School and founder and director of the Arizona Center for Integrative Medicine at the University of Arizona, where he is a professor of medicine and public health.

Andrew Weil, *Why Our Health Matters: A Vision of Medicine That Can Transform Our Future*. New York: Hudson Street, 2009.

The British system is considered by most health care experts to be the most cost-efficient system in the world. Because it does not need to pay for marketing or billing, for example, the administrative costs are very low. In addition, doctors are paid a set fee for each patient, rather than a fee for each visit with a patient, so this limits doctor fees. It also creates a built-in incentive for doctors to emphasize preventive care; doctors want to keep their patients as healthy as possible so that they do not come in for many appointments. However, the NHS is a massive operation, and the taxes required to pay for it are high. Many people complain that they must first see their primary doctor before they can schedule an appointment with a specialist, and about the long waits to see specialists or get surgery. The NHS also controls costs by refusing to pay for some tests, procedures, and medications—a feature that many people criticize as rationing. Because of these and other criticisms, Britain is planning to overhaul the NHS in the near future. The system will be reorganized to provide local doctors with more control over medical services. Britain also has a small private insurance sector and private health facilities where patients can pay out of pocket or with private insurance if they are denied NHS services or choose not to take advantage of the NHS system.

France—The Best Health Care in the World?

Although Britain ranks high in terms of overall costs, according to the World Health Organization (WHO), France's health care system—considered a variation of the Bismarck model—offers the best health care in the world. In a 2000 report that reviewed health care systems around the world, WHO ranked the French system first. WHO said that France's health care excelled in four areas: overall health of the population; universal coverage; responsive health care providers; and freedom of choice for patients.

PROBLEMS WITH U.S. PRIVATE HEALTH INSURANCE

"Private insurers [in the United States] . . . seek out the healthy and leave the ill uninsured or scrambling to qualify for shrinking public programs."—John Geyman, author and professor of family medicine at the University of Washington School of Medicine in Seattle.

John Geyman, "The Common Interest: Is It Time for National Health Insurance?" *Boston Review*, November/December 2005. http://bostonreview.net/BR30.6/geyman.php.

The French adopted their comprehensive, universal government-run health insurance program in 1945 during a postwar economic boom and funded it largely with taxes on employees. The French system is part of the country's social

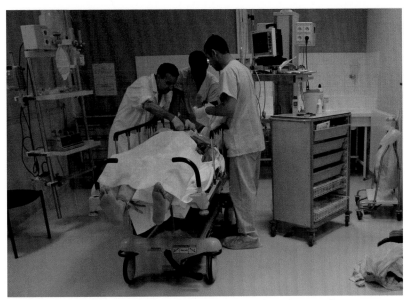

Doctors treat a patient in an emergency ward in France. The French system, a variation of the Bismarck Model, is touted as the best in the world by the World Health Organization.

insurance program, and it resembles America's Medicare system except that it covers everyone, with no deductibles. Every person legally in France is entitled to basic health care coverage under this program, and the government pays for health insurance to cover the unemployed. In addition, private insurance is available to cover out-of-pocket co-payments, dental and eye care, and extra amenities like private hospital rooms. As in the United States, the French system relies on private medical providers, giving patients complete freedom to choose their doctors. However, compared with U.S. Medicare, the French health care benefits are very generous. As *Bloomberg Businessweek* reports:

> In France, the sicker you get, the less you pay. Chronic diseases, such as diabetes, and critical surgeries, such as a coronary bypass, are reimbursed at 100%. Cancer patients are treated free of charge. Patients suffering from colon cancer, for instance, can receive Genentech Inc.'s Avastin [a prescription medication] without charge. In the U.S., a patient may pay $48,000 a year.[32]

The cost of the French health care system is more than Britain's but still much less than the overall cost of U.S. health care. France is able to keep its costs low partly because it pays doctors and other providers much less than what doctors earn in the United States; on the other hand, French doctors have their medical school costs and social security taxes paid for by the government, and malpractice insurance rates are low. Despite the system's success, France, like all other countries, has been challenged in recent years by ever-rising health care costs. In response, the government has reduced the reimbursement rate for many prescriptions and medical services—a decision that has raised co-payments and created more opportunity for private insurers to sell policies to cover the gap.

Canada's Experience with a Public Plan

Canada's health care is a mixed Bismarck/Beverage system. First developed in the 1960s, it is publicly funded, administered by the government in a decentralized manner under government guidelines, and paid for by income and sales taxes. The system covers all Canadians regardless of preexisting conditions or income, with no co-payments or deductibles, and it usually provides preventive care, medical treatments, dental surgery, and a range of other services. Prescription drugs are typically covered only for the elderly and the poor, but drug prices are kept low because the government negotiates prices with drug suppliers. Individual provinces in Canada each develop their own health care budgets and administer the national health care program, but services are provided by private doctors and private, mostly nonprofit hospitals. Unlike the U.S. system, Canada's system is not employer-based. However, as in America, Canada also has a system of private insurance companies. In Canada, however, private insurers are not permitted to offer plans for basic health care. Canadian insurers are limited to covering benefits not offered by the public plan, such as routine dentistry, prescription drugs, auto accidents, care while traveling abroad, cosmetic procedures, and private hospital rooms.

In general, most commentators agree that the majority of Canadians like their health care system. In Canada, people

Prescription Drugs from Canada

The high prices of prescription drugs in the United States have led many Americans to consider buying their prescriptions in Canada, where costs are significantly lower. The main reason that prescription medications are cheaper in Canada is related largely to Canada's government-run health care system. The Canadian government sets a maximum market price on all brand name drugs sold in Canada and then allows those prices to rise only at the rate of inflation. In addition, in each of Canada's provinces, health plan regulators develop a list of drugs that will be paid for under the plan, which enables them to negotiate lower prices for some of the most popular medications. These government regulatory actions limit the amount that drug companies can charge pharmacies and other distributors of drugs, reduce the price gap between brand name and generic drugs, and protect consumers from price gouging by drug companies.

Some commentators argue, however, that this type of foreign regulation of drugs encourages drug companies to charge excessive prices in the United States, the only nation that does not have price controls, to make up for losses elsewhere. Americans thus subsidize prescription drugs for Canada and other countries. Under U.S. law, importing drugs from Canada is illegal, but the U.S. Food and Drug Administration typically does not prosecute Americans who buy up to a three-month supply of Canadian medications for personal use. As a result, many Americans are purchasing medications from online Canadian pharmacies or driving over the border to pick them up in person.

New Hampshire governor Craig Benson, left, shows seniors how to buy prescription drugs from Canada on the Internet. Out of economic necessity many Americans are getting prescription drugs through Canada.

have access to quality care when they need it and do not go bankrupt trying to pay medical bills. However, Canadians have complained about long waits to see specialists or to have certain types of procedures. In the 1990s Canada's Supreme Court even found that some patients had died as a result of waiting for medical procedures. The government responded by providing funding to eliminate wait times for some of the most urgent procedures, such as cancer care, cardiac care, and joint replacement operations. According to some reports, however, the waits are still long—up to seventeen weeks—to see specialists or to get nonurgent procedures such as colonoscopies.

Comparing U.S. Health Care with Other Countries

During recent health care debates, conservatives have often raised fears about reforms that would make the U.S. health care system more like systems in Europe or Canada, calling them socialized medicine that sacrifice the quality of care and freedom of choice available in America. These critics typically point to the wait times for medical services in Britain and Canada and claim that health care will be rationed under any type of government-run system. Proponents of reform, on the other hand, sometimes offer unconditional praise for many of the foreign health care programs, claiming they provide superior health care and urging U.S. policy makers to adopt a similar program for America. Controversial film maker Michael Moore, for example, released a documentary in 2007 called *Sicko*, which emphasizes the many virtues of the government-run health care systems in France, England, Canada, and Cuba, while completely vilifying U.S. health care.

An independent review of the world's health care systems in 2000 by the World Health Organization (WHO), a United Nations health agency, ranked the United States far behind most other developed countries in the quality of its medical care. As the WHO report concluded, "The U.S. health system spends a higher portion of its gross domestic product than any other country but ranks 37 out of 191 countries according to its performance."[33] WHO's assessment is based on five indicators:

overall health of each country's population; health inequalities; the responsiveness of health care providers to patient needs; how well people in all economic categories are served by the system; and whether the costs of care are fairly distributed across the population served. WHO found that the U.S. health care system is very responsive but ranks low in other categories, such as equality of care, providing care to those with less money, and financing care fairly.

AMERICANS HAPPY WITH THEIR HEALTH CARE

"More than eight in 10 [Americans] . . . are satisfied with the quality of care they now receive and relatively content with their own current expenses."—Ceci Connolly and Jon Cohen, staff writers for the *Washington Post*, a daily newspaper based in Washington, D.C.

Ceci Connolly and Jon Cohen, "Most Want Health Reform but Fear Its Side Effects," *Washington Post*, June 24, 2009. www.washingtonpost.com/wp-dyn/content/article/2009/06/23/AR2009062303510.html.

A more recent study by the Commonwealth Fund, a private health care research group in the United States, examines the quality of health care in five countries—the United States, Britain, Canada, Germany, and Australia—using surveys of patients and doctors and analysis of other data. Its report, issued in May 2007, ranks America last or next-to-last on many measures of performance. For example, the report finds that all other industrialized nations provide universal care while many people in the United States lack adequate insurance coverage. The United States also ranks last in providing equitable care, since it has the greatest disparity in the quality of care provided to richer versus poorer Americans. And Americans are less healthy than people in other industrialized countries in certain categories; compared with other industrialized nations, the United States has a high infant mortality rate, lower healthy life expectancy, and a terrible obesity epidemic. In overall quality, the United States is rated last, with poor scores for coordinating the care of chronically ill patients, meeting patient needs, and avoiding fatal surgical or medical mistakes. The one area in which the United States ranks high is in providing the right care according to standard clinical guidelines, especially preventive care like Pap smears and mammograms to detect early-stage cancers.

A 2010 update by the Commonwealth Fund finds that not much has changed; it concludes:

> Despite having the most costly health system in the world, the United States consistently underperforms on most dimensions of performance, relative to other countries. . . . Compared with six other nations—Australia, Canada, Germany, the Netherlands, New Zealand, and the United Kingdom—the U.S. health care system ranks last or next-to-last on five dimensions of a high performance health system: quality, access, efficiency, equity, and healthy lives.[34]

At the same time, no country's health care system is perfect, and all systems have room for improvement. As a 2001 analysis by the Heritage Foundation, a conservative think tank, points out, problems are evident in many European health care systems. These include lack of competition among providers, limited choice of doctors, long waits for medical services, and rising health care costs for governments. Even France, considered to have the world's best health care system by many experts, faces challenges. For example, according to French newsmagazine editor Philippe Manière:

> Universal coverage [in France] does not mean universal access to quality care [because] . . . the result of France's guarantee [of health care to all] is a cash-strapped system riddled with abuse. [In addition, the French health care system shows that] . . . making across-the-board price cuts on pharmaceuticals to save money can have adverse effects. In France, such cuts tend to restrict research and development and to reduce the availability of cutting edge drugs, while other areas of medicine requiring significant reform are overlooked.[35]

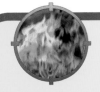

Michael Moore's Movie *Sicko*

In 2007 American documentary film-maker Michael Moore released a controversial film called *Sicko* that focuses on the problems in the U.S. health care system. *Sicko* compares the U.S. for-profit health insurance industry with the nonprofit health care systems in Britain, France, Canada, and Cuba. Although the film was sharply criticized for making foreign health care systems appear to be too perfect, it is nevertheless compelling because it features interviews with Americans who have health insurance but are in financial debt due to the high cost of insurance co-payments, surgery, and prescription medication. Also, Moore features rescue workers who volunteered after the September 11, 2001, terrorist attacks, and who subsequently developed medical problems that they could not afford to treat in the United States; the group travels to Cuba where they receive free or inexpensive medical treatment. Many commentators praised Moore's main message—that

people have nothing to fear from a government-run health care system—and argued that his critique of the U.S. for-profit insurance industry was completely accurate. Others, however, criticized Moore for his theatrics and for failing to investigate the problems in foreign health care systems. The film was nominated for an Academy Award for Documentary Feature and is now available in DVD format.

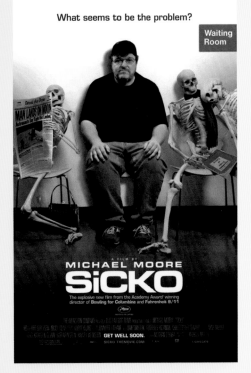

American documentary filmmaker Michael Moore released Sicko *in 2007. It was a scathing indictment of America's health care system and was very controversial.*

The European system most admired by conservative experts is Switzerland's—a universal system enacted in 1994 that is based on private insurance purchased by individuals, with government subsidies for the poor. Premiums are not based on health risks or income; they are set according to each person's age, sex, and location. The system works through a risk-adjustment system in which all insurers pay into a central fund and then are provided assistance from the fund according to the number of high-risk patients they insure. Insurers are required to offer basic health services on a nonprofit basis, but otherwise, they are free to design benefits packages and charge whatever they want. Typically, most insurers charge co-payments for medical services as well as a yearly deductible, and Swiss law prohibits patients from insuring against co-payments in most cases. This system is designed to encourage citizens to rely on private savings for a significant portion of their health care—a goal that supporters say causes patients to make more informed health care decisions and pursue preventive care and lifestyles in order to avoid future health risks. Yet Switzerland, too, has its critics who complain that its health care is not equitable, since everyone pays the same premiums regardless of income, and that rising health costs are making it very expensive for many families as well as for the government.

No country, therefore, has developed a health care system that suits everyone. But it is against this background of many different, but all less-than-perfect health care options that U.S. policy makers have been challenged to develop a health care system that works for America.

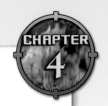

THE PATIENT PROTECTION AND AFFORDABLE CARE ACT

The most recent attempt to reform America's health care system was made by President Barack Obama in 2009 and 2010—an effort that led to the passage of the Patient Protection and Affordable Care Act (PPACA), also more simply called the Affordable Care Act (ACA), on March 23, 2010. Obama signaled his support for health care reform even before he was elected and made the issue one of his first priorities once he became president. The process of passing the legislation was prolonged and extremely difficult, with strong opposition from both Republicans in Congress and lobbyists for the insurance industry, but health experts agree that the result was historic—universal health care for almost all Americans achieved through mandates on both employers and individuals, with government subsidies to make health insurance affordable. However, the new law remains controversial, and opponents have promised to fight its implementation.

Health Care Costs Balloon

During the first decade of the new millennium, U.S. health care costs continued to balloon out of control. As of 2006, a federal report found that annual U.S. health care spending already totaled $2.2 trillion, or $7,421 per person. Despite a deep recession, health care costs jumped again in the next couple of years. By 2008 government reports disclosed that U.S. health care spending had grown to $2.3 trillion, or $7,681 per person—a record 16.2 percent of the U.S. economy. According to experts,

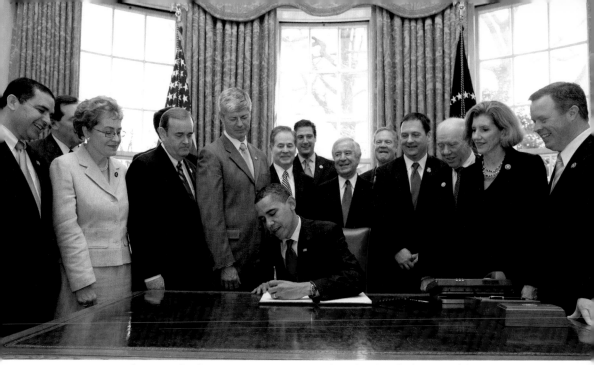

President Barack Obama signs an executive order related to the passing of the Patient Protection and Affordable Care Act in March 2010.

this is twice the average cost of health care in other developed countries. Rising costs affect both government Medicare/Medicaid spending as well as individual families. In fact, average family health care premiums have more than doubled since 2000—from $6,800 in 2000 to $12,700 in 2008—and these steadily rising premiums, combined with higher deductibles and fewer benefits, are the main reason that growing numbers of people are opting to go without any type of health insurance. Not surprisingly, health reform thus became a central issue in the 2008 presidential campaigns.

In fact, all the presidential candidates for the November 2008 presidential election promised health care reform, but Republican and Democratic proposals had major differences. Republican candidates Senator John McCain, New York City mayor Rudolph Giuliani, former Arkansas governor Mike Huckabee, and former Massachusetts governor Mitt Romney generally proposed to increase insurance coverage for individuals through new tax incentives and deregulation of state insurance markets. The Democratic candidates, Senator Barack Obama, Senator Hillary Clinton, and Senator John Edwards, however, promised more sweeping reforms.

Obama's campaign, for example, pledged to create a new national health plan to cover most Americans and provide affordable health coverage similar to the comprehensive insurance provided to members of Congress. Obama said that he would accomplish this by requiring employers either to provide health care to employees or pay a penalty, and by establishing a government-run National Health Insurance Exchange to help self-employed and other individuals purchase affordable insurance. Obama's goals also included curbing insurance company abuses and cutting health care costs. Impressed with Obama's proposal, on January 28, 2008, Senator Edward Kennedy, a longtime Democratic crusader for universal health care, endorsed Obama's campaign, stating, "With Barack Obama, we will break the old gridlock and finally make health care what it should be in America—a fundamental right for all, not just an expensive privilege for the few."[36]

AN EXPANSION OF HEALTH CARE COVERAGE

"The Affordable Care Act is not a magic pill that will cure all the problems in our health care system. . . . But this law is the biggest expansion in health care coverage since Medicare." —Kathleen Sebelius, U.S. secretary of health and human services.

Kathleen Sebelius, "Sebelius Remarks: Health Reform and You: How the New Law Will Increase Your Health Security," HHS.gov, April 6, 2010. www.hhs.gov/news/press/2010pres/04/20100406b.html.

After he was elected, Obama made health care reform a high priority. He named Kansas governor Kathleen Sebelius as secretary of health and human services to lead the administration's health reform efforts, and in March 2009 he held a White House health care forum, pledging to get a health care plan passed by the end of 2009. However, instead of submitting Obama's own bill to the legislature, the White House allowed Congress to develop its own legislation, and months passed with little progress and heavy partisan conflict. Finally, in a September 9, 2009, speech to Congress, Obama outlined the details of his basic plan for health care reform and asked Congress for quick action. He stated:

> The plan I'm announcing tonight would meet three basic goals: It will provide more security and stability to those who have health insurance. It will provide insurance to those who don't. And it will slow the growth of health care costs for our families, our businesses, and our government. It's a plan that asks everyone to take responsibility for meeting this challenge—not just government and insurance companies, but employers and individuals. . . .
>
> Here are the details that every American needs to know about this plan: First, if you are among the hundreds of millions of Americans who already have health insurance through your job, Medicare, Medicaid, or the VA, nothing in this plan will require you or your employer to change the coverage or the doctor you have. . . . Under this plan, it will be against the law for insurance companies to deny you coverage because of a pre-existing condition. As soon as I sign this bill, it will be against the law for insurance companies to drop your coverage when you get sick or water it down when you need it most. They will no longer be able to place some arbitrary cap on the amount of coverage you can receive in a given year or a lifetime. We will place a limit on how much you can be charged for out-of-pocket expenses, because in the United States of America, no one should go broke because they get sick. And insurance companies will be required to cover, with no extra charge, routine check-ups and preventive care, like mammograms and colonoscopies—because there's no reason we shouldn't be catching diseases like breast cancer and colon cancer before they get worse. That makes sense, it saves money, and it saves lives. . . .
>
> Now, if you're one of the tens of millions of Americans who don't currently have health insurance, the second part of this plan will finally offer you quality, affordable

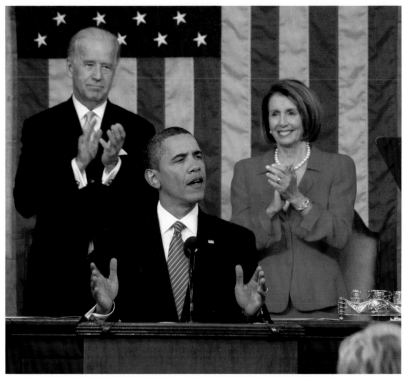

In a speech to a joint session of Congress on September 9, 2009, President Barack Obama outlined the details of his basic plan for health care reform.

choices. If you lose your job or change your job, you will be able to get coverage. If you strike out on your own and start a small business, you will be able to get coverage. We will do this by creating a new insurance exchange— a marketplace where individuals and small businesses will be able to shop for health insurance at competitive prices. Insurance companies will have an incentive to participate in this exchange because it lets them compete for millions of new customers. As one big group, these customers will have greater leverage to bargain with the insurance companies for better prices and quality coverage. . . . For those individuals and small businesses who still cannot afford the lower-priced insurance available in the exchange, we will provide tax credits, the size of which will be based on your need. . . . This exchange will take effect in four years, which will give us time to do it right. In the meantime, for those Americans who can't get insurance today because they have pre-existing medical conditions, we will immediately offer low-cost coverage that will protect you against financial ruin if you become seriously ill. . . .

[U]nder my plan, individuals will be required to carry basic health insurance—just as most states require you to carry auto insurance. Likewise, businesses will be required to either offer their workers health care, or chip in to help cover the cost of their workers. There will be a hardship waiver for those individuals who still cannot afford coverage, and 95% of all small businesses, because of their size and narrow profit margin, would be exempt from these requirements. . . . But we cannot have large businesses and individuals who can afford coverage game the system by avoiding responsibility to themselves or their employees. Improving our health care system only works if everybody does their part.[37]

On November 7, 2009, the House of Representatives passed its version of health care reform by a narrow 220-215 vote, with many Democrats voting against the bill and only one Republican voting for it. This was followed by Senate approval of its health care reform bill on December 24, 2009, with all sixty Senate Democrats voting for the bill and all Republicans voting against it. Senate Democratic leaders were able to achieve the required sixty-vote majority needed to prevent Republicans from filibustering (or blocking) the bill only by making a much-criticized deal with Democratic Nebraska senator Ben Nelson, exempting his state from certain Medicaid costs included in the bill.

But these successes were followed by months of disagreements between legislators about the details of the final version of the legislation. In large part, this delay occurred because a Republican, Scott Brown, won a special Senate election in Massachusetts to replace longtime Democratic senator Edward Kennedy, who died of cancer in 2009. Brown's win left Senate Democrats without the sixty votes needed to pass a final bill.

Senator Edward Kennedy's Fight for Universal Health Care

Senator Edward Kennedy, a Democratic senator from Massachusetts for forty-seven years, was one of the nation's most committed fighters for universal health care. He was first elected to the Senate in 1962 and soon became chairman of the powerful Senate Committee on Health, Education, Labor, and Pensions. Throughout his career, "Ted" Kennedy worked tirelessly to expand access and improve the quality of health care. Although he was unsuccessful during his lifetime in passing a universal health care bill, he came close in 1974 when he agreed to work with Republican president Richard Nixon to pass the administration's Comprehensive Health Insurance Act—a law that never was enacted due to the crisis created by Nixon's Watergate scandal. However, Kennedy was instrumental in passing a list of other health-related initiatives, including important laws such as the Consolidated Omnibus Budget Reconciliation Act of 1986 (COBRA), which provides temporary health insurance coverage for the unemployed; the 1986 Emergency Medical Treatment and Active Labor Act (EMTALA), which prohibits hospitals from turning away emergency patients because they have no health insurance;

and the Health Insurance Portability and Accountability Act (HIPAA) of 1996, a law that guarantees that people can change jobs and insurers without being penalized for preexisting conditions. In addition, Kennedy helped enact the 1997 Children's Health Insurance Program, which provides insurance coverage to children in low- and moderate-income families, and the Medicare Modernization Act of 2003, which provides for Medicare prescription drug coverage. Kennedy died on August 25, 2009, before President Obama's health care reform bill was passed by Congress, but many commentators say that it was Kennedy who paved the way for this victory.

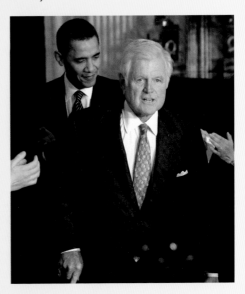

In his forty-seven years in the U.S. Senate Ted Kennedy worked tirelessly for universal health care until his death in August 2009.

Many political commentators even thought health care reform was dead at this point. Finally, following a tense bipartisan summit between lawmakers and the president in February 2010, a compromise bill was passed on March 21, 2010, by the House and followed by Senate approval. In a festive ceremony at the White House on March 23, 2010, Obama signed the landmark reform legislation, saying that it achieved "the core principle that everybody should have some basic security when it comes to their health care."[38]

A Bitter Process

Although ultimately successful, the process of enacting the legislation was contentious and highly partisan. The American Medical Association (AMA) endorsed the ACA, and little opposition came from doctors, hospitals, or insurance companies, but there was a prolonged political battle between Democrats and Republicans over core issues, with Republican claims that the reforms would create "death panels" and lead to "socialized medicine."[39]

STRANGULATION OF PRIVATE HEALTH INSURANCE

"The new health care legislation is a step toward elimination, by slow strangulation, of private health insurance and establishment of government as the 'single payer.'"—George Will, a weekly columnist for the *Washington Post*, an American newspaper.

George Will, "Let Us Disclose That Free-Speech Limits Are Harmful," *Washington Post*, July 11, 2010. www.washingtonpost.com/wp-dyn/content/article/2010/07/09/AR2010070903806.html.

One of the fiercest fights concerned whether the health care bill should contain a public option—that is, a government-run insurance program that patients could choose instead of private health care insurance. Many Democrats strongly pushed for this idea, believing that a public insurance option would provide much-needed competition for private insurers and an

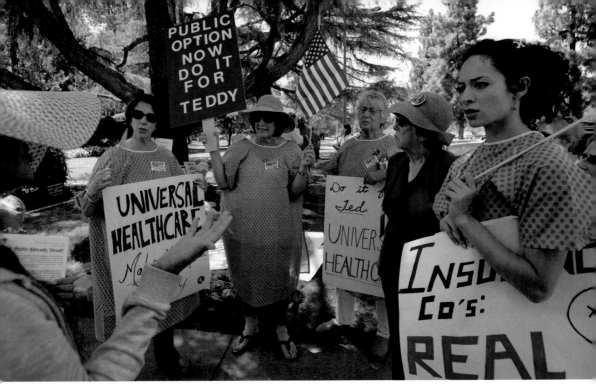

The debate over the public option split the country along party lines, and from the halls of Congress to town hall meetings there was bitter debate.

effective way to control costs and stop insurance abuses. Opponents, mainly Republicans, vehemently disagreed. They said that cheaper premiums under a public option would likely attract so many people that the government would become too powerful, able to drive down insurance premiums to the point that private insurers would no longer be able to compete. Ultimately, opponents warned, the public option would evolve into a Medicare-for-all system that could put private insurers out of business and give the government broad control over individual medical decisions. As Karen Ignagni, president of an insurance industry lobby group, puts it, "It's a very short step [from a public option] to a Medicare-like program for all Americans in a single-payer system."[40]

In the end, in order to get Senate approval for a compromise health care reform bill, Senate Democrats agreed to drop the public option from their version of the legislation. Another compromise, this one made by House Democrats at the very end of the legislative process, was a deal with opponents of abortion rights that involved Obama issuing an executive order to ensure that federal money provided by the bill could not be used for abortions. This agreement helped House Democrats secure the last few Democratic votes needed to pass the final bill. Even with these compromises, the legislation passed in the House without a single Republican vote.

Reforms Contained in the Bill

Although not a radical plan, the ACA's package of reforms was nevertheless historic. As Robert Reich, a former U.S. secretary of labor and now professor of public policy at the University of California at Berkeley, explains: "It's not nearly as momentous as the passage of Medicare in 1965 and won't fundamentally alter how Americans think about social safety nets. But the passage of Obama's healthcare reform bill is the biggest thing Congress has done in decades, and [it] has enormous political significance for the future."[41] The Congressional Budget Office (CBO), for example, estimates that the law will provide health coverage to an additional 32 million currently uninsured Americans. And although the basic structure of America's health care system—employer-based health care insurance provided by private insurance companies—is retained, the law also ends some of the most egregious practices of health insurance companies and attempts to lower health costs through a variety of incentives and changes.

A GOVERNMENT-FIRST LAW

"Obamacare is a hastily crafted maze of Washington-empowering, government-first policies that will forever scar the quality, affordability and accessibility of health care in this nation."—Tom Price, a Republican congressman from Georgia.

Tom Price, "Price: U.S. Health Care Will Be Scarred," *Roll Call*, June 21, 2010. www .rollcall.com/features/Health-Care-Next-Steps_2010/health_care/47486-1.html.

The law is structured, however, to take effect very slowly. Initially, most Americans will see only very minor changes, with the biggest changes happening in 2014. Still, the ACA ends certain insurer practices almost immediately. For example, in 2010 it requires that children with preexisting conditions be covered and that dependent children under the age of twenty-six be allowed to remain on their parents' health insurance policies. Also in 2010, insurance companies are prohibited from rescinding health insurance once subscribers become ill, prevented from imposing lifetime or unreasonable yearly limits on benefits, required to implement a new process for appealing benefit denials, and required to provide coverage for preventive services on new plans without co-pays (and on all plans by 2018). In addition,

Rationing Health Care

One of the arguments against health care reform is that it will lead to rationing of medical care. Supporters of reform, however, often argue that the U.S. health care system—that is, the private insurance industry—already rations care by denying care to those who cannot afford to pay for it. In the future, however, soaring health care costs, exacerbated by factors such as the rapidly aging U.S. population, may cause the United States to eventually adopt some sort of formal rationing system. In fact, end-of-life care consumes the largest part of the Medicare budget—$55 billion in 2009. Seventy-five percent of all Americans die in a hospital, many of them in intensive care, where they are attended by multiple doctors and specialists and subjected to a battery of expensive high-tech tests and procedures. This end-of-life care can easily cost $10,000 per day. Many people say these efforts often do not extend life, can infringe on the quality of life in patients' last days, and can leave taxpayers with exorbitant bills.

Conservatives argue that the Affordable Care Act's (ACA) creation of an Independent Payment Advisory Board (IPAB)—a Medicare cost-cutting measure—is a first step toward government rationing. The ACA establishes specific target growth rates for Medicare and charges the IPAB with ensuring that Medicare expenditures stay within these limits. ACA supporters, however, point out that the ACA specifically prohibits the IPAB from including recommendations to ration health care, raise revenues, raise Medicare beneficiary premiums, increase Medicare beneficiary cost-sharing, or otherwise restrict benefits or modify eligibility criteria. The question of rationing, therefore, is one that might not arise immediately, but perhaps one that must be addressed in the future.

beginning in 2010, adults with preexisting conditions will be able to buy coverage through expanded high-risk insurance pools set up by the government. And the act requires a $250 rebate in 2010 to seniors to help them pay for prescription drugs not covered by Medicare. This gap in Medicare's prescription coverage, often referred to as the "doughnut hole," will be completely closed by 2020. Other immediate changes include a 10 percent tax on indoor tanning services and tax credits for businesses with fewer than 50 employees to cover 35 percent of their health care premiums (increasing to 50 percent by 2014).

A PRESCRIPTION FOR HIGHER COSTS

"The PPACA . . . is a prescription for ever growing health care costs possibly even beyond that which would have occurred absent the legislation."—R.D. Quinn, a retired corporate executive who blogs about various issues on the website Quinn's Commentary.

R.D. Quinn, "Why the Patient Protection Affordable Care Act (PPACA) Will Not Produce the Stated Savings . . . and Why You Should Care," April 29, 2010. http://quinnscommentary.com/2010/04/29/why-the-patient-protection-affordable-care-act-ppaca-will-not-produce-the-stated-savings-and-why-you-should-care.

In 2011 a number of other changes will be implemented, many of them affecting Medicare. For example, Medicare will cover annual wellness visits and personalized prevention plans, a 50 percent discount will be provided on brand-name drugs for seniors along with other future drug discounts, and the Medicare payroll tax will increase from 1.45 percent to 2.35 percent for individuals earning more than $200,000 (and married couples filing jointly earning above $250,000). The government also will help ease the administrative burdens on small businesses that offer health insurance benefits and will require insurers to spend at least 80–85 percent of premium dollars on direct medical care and efforts to improve the quality of care.

In 2013 the bill requires health insurers to begin implementing standards for the electronic exchange of health information in order to reduce paperwork and administrative costs. Also in 2013, among other changes, government subsidies for Medicare Part D (Medicare Advantage) will be eliminated to help pay for the new law.

The ACA produces its most far-reaching changes in 2014. At this point, businesses with 50 or more employees must offer coverage to employees or pay a $2,000 penalty per employee. Moreover, insurers will no longer be permitted to refuse coverage to adults who have preexisting health conditions, and they cannot charge higher rates because of heath status, gender, or other factors. In addition, all Americans will be required to purchase basic health insurance or pay a fine ($95 in 2014, $325 in 2015, $695 or up to 2.5 percent of income in 2016), although exceptions will be given for financial hardship. Also, the act requires states to contract with private insurers to create multistate health insurance exchanges to help individuals and small employers shop for affordable plans. In addition, Medicaid will be expanded to cover people whose income is up to 133 percent of the poverty level. People who are poor but whose income is above Medicaid levels will receive subsidies to help them purchase insurance. And these are just some of the most significant reforms; the number of changes made by the act are too numerous to discuss in detail.

All of this will be paid for by the changes in Medicare and by a tax that will take effect in 2018 on people who have so-called Cadillac plans—employer-provided health insurance plans of more than $27,500 for family coverage and $10,200 for single coverage. Also, the government will impose new fees on drug manufacturers, health insurance companies, and medical device manufacturers.

Criticisms of the New Law

Following the passage of ACA, many reform advocates hailed the legislation for making a fundamental, positive change in U.S. health care. *New York Times* journalist David Leonhardt, for example, praised the new law for improving equity, saying, "The [ACA] . . . is the federal government's biggest attack on economic inequality since inequality began rising more than three decades

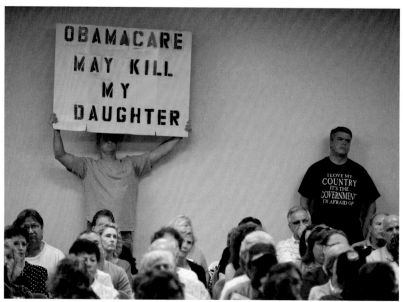

Many Republicans complained that "Obamacare" would increase costs, expand Medicaid, and cause millions to lose their employer-provided health care.

ago. . . . The bill . . . aims to smooth out one of the roughest edges in American society—the inability of many people to afford medical care after they lose a job or get sick. And it would do so in large measure by taxing the rich."[42]

However, criticism also continued from both the political left and the right. Democrats who wanted to see a public option or a single-payer system similar to Medicare lamented that the new law failed to achieve this goal. In a July 29, 2010, statement, for example, U.S. representatives Dennis Kucinich (D-Ohio), John Conyers (Michigan), and U.S. senator Bernie Sanders (Vermont) argued that a Medicare-for-all health care system in the United States still has substantial support and vowed to continue their push for such a program, stating, "We believe that Medicare for All is inevitable in the United States. It is up to all of us to determine when the inevitable becomes the reality."[43]

Many Republicans, meanwhile, complained that Obama's health care reforms, which they nicknamed "Obamacare," will increase costs, expand Medicaid, cause millions of people to lose their employer-provided health care, and give the federal government unprecedented control over health care. As Kevin Hasset, director of economic policy studies at the American Enterprise Institute, a conservative think tank, argues,

> A sprawling, complex bureaucracy has been set up that will have almost absolute power to dictate terms for participating in the health-care system. That's what the law does to government. What it does to [consumers] . . . is worse. Based on the administration's own numbers, as many as 117 million people might have to change their health plans by 2013 as their employer-provided coverage loses its grandfathered status and becomes subject to the new Obamacare mandates. Those mandates also might make . . . health care more expensive. The Congressional Budget Office predicts that premiums for . . . families who buy their insurance privately will rise by as much as $2,100. The central Obamacare mechanism for increasing insurance coverage is an expansion of the Medicaid program. Of the 30 million new people covered, 16 million will be enrolled in Medicaid.[44]

President Obama and his health and human services secretary, Kathleen Sebelius (in pink), went on the road to many town hall meetings explaining his health care reform.

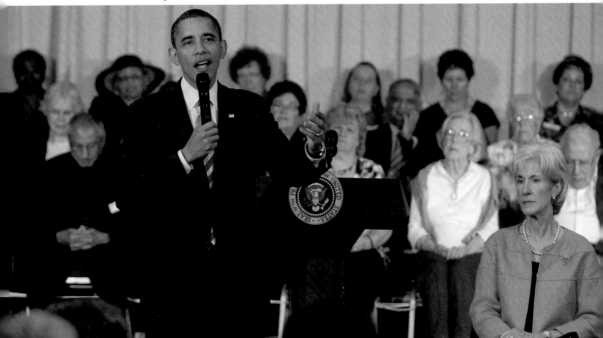

Many Americans agreed with this assessment. According to a *USA Today*/Gallup poll conducted shortly after the ACA was enacted, almost two-thirds of Americans said that the new law costs too much and expands the government's role in health care too far.

Responding to his critics, Obama strongly defended his health care plan, touting its benefits for consumers. In remarks on June 22, 2009, the president said:

> This law will cut costs and make coverage more afford-able for families and small businesses. . . . It's reform that finally extends the opportunity to purchase coverage to the millions who currently don't have it—and includes tough new consumer protections to guarantee greater stability, security and control for the millions who do have health insurance. . . . Individuals and small businesses will finally have the same access to the same types of insurance plans that members of Congress have for themselves.[45]

Only time will tell whether Obama's critics or his supporters are correct, but some commentators have noted that an earlier health care reform—called Medicare—also was bitterly attacked in the months after it was enacted; yet it became one of the nation's most popular social programs.

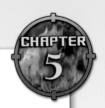

THE FUTURE OF
U.S. HEALTH CARE

In the months following March 23, 2010, enactment of the Patient Protection and Affordable Care Act, policy makers, insurers, medical providers, and the public were faced with the task of trying to understand its complex provisions, mandates, and effective dates. Significant opposition to Obama's health care legislation lingered, most notably evidenced in Republican calls for repeal and lawsuits filed by states seeking to overturn the new law as unconstitutional. Assuming the law is upheld in the courts and not repealed by the Congress, however, many political commentators think that public acceptance will increase over the next several years as the ACA slowly takes effect and people begin realizing its benefits. The real questions, according to health care experts, are how the bill will affect health care in the United States over the long run and how the U.S. health care system might further evolve in the future.

Efforts to Repeal or Limit
the Affordable Care Act

The controversy surrounding the ACA did not end when it was signed into law. Soon after its passage, many Republican lawmakers served notice that they would campaign on a pledge to repeal the ACA in the fall 2010 midterm congressional elections. Senator Jim DeMint, a Republican from South Carolina, introduced legislation in Congress to accomplish this goal of repeal, explaining,

> Unless this trillion-dollar assault on our freedoms is repealed, it will force Americans to purchase Washington-approved health plans or face stiff penalties. It will fund

abortions, raise taxes and insurance premiums, while reducing health care choices and quality. . . . This arrogant power grab proves that the President and his party care more about government control than the will of the American people.[46]

Also, immediately after the ACA's enactment, a total of twenty-one states filed suit in federal court claiming that the law violates the U.S. Constitution's commerce clause by requiring nearly all Americans to purchase health insurance. Other legal arguments in the lawsuits claim that the federal reform violates states rights guaranteed by the Tenth Amendment, by requiring states to administer and support the law's expansion of health care and by making the federal government too powerful in the area of health care. The litigating states include Florida, Arizona, Alabama, Colorado, Idaho, Louisiana, Michigan, Nebraska, Pennsylvania, South Carolina, South Dakota, Texas, Utah, Washington, Virginia, Indiana, North Dakota, Mississippi, Nevada, Georgia, and Alaska.

Republican senators Jim DeMint (S.C.), right, and Tom Coburn (Okla.), at the lectern, outline their plans to the press on with their efforts to repeal the Affordable Care Act.

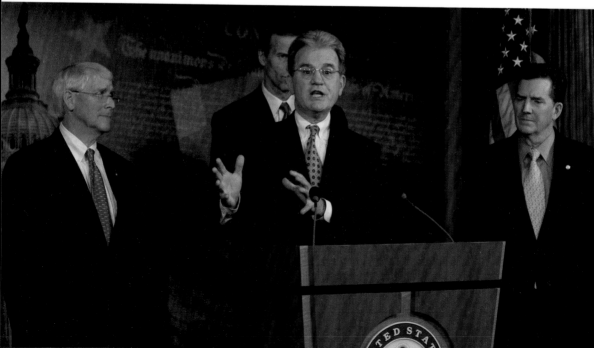

In addition, some thirty-eight states have introduced legislation called the Freedom of Choice in Health Care Act—model legislation proposed by the American Legislative Exchange Council (ALEC), a national association of conservative state legislators. The bills would block the federal ACA's imposition of penalties on individuals who fail to purchase health insurance, thereby forcing a showdown with the federal government.

INSURANCE INDUSTRY PROFITS

"Insurance 'reforms' [in the ACA] won't prevent insurers from . . . maximizing their own profits as their underinsurance products become ever less adequate. . . . They have wide latitude to set their premium rates despite the concerns of regulators. [And] plans can still deny coverage or even cancel policies."—John Geyman, a professor of family medicine at the University of Washington School of Medicine in Seattle.

John Geyman, "Hijacked: Stolen Health Reform III: How Much Will Access to Care Be Expanded?" Physicians for a National Health Program, July 15, 2010. http://pnhp.org/blog/2010/07/15/hijacked-stolen-health-reform-iii-how-much-will-access-to-care-be-expanded.

Conservatives are counting on either the courts or the Congress to overturn health care reforms. If the ACA survives these attacks, however, many other commentators predict that the American public will eventually understand its benefits and accept the reforms, especially once the law takes full effect in 2014. Pointing to polls showing growing support for the ACA, Maggie Mahar of the the Century Foundation, a progressive think tank, argues:

> [In March 2010], few Americans knew what was in the 2,500 page bill, or what impact it would have on their lives. Uncertainty fueled anxiety. But with each passing week, the public learns more about health care reform. . . . The more Americans learn about the details of the legislation, and how reform will help them and their families, the better they will like it.[47]

Early Implementation of the Affordable Care Act

In the summer of 2010, Obama's administration worked to ease the anxiety surrounding the ACA and implement the law's early health care reforms. Sebelius sent a letter to congressional leaders in early May 2010 outlining the government's initial steps. One first step involved issuing regulations to implement new insurance mandates. And the secretary announced that the insurance industry agreed to early implementation of two provisions of the ACA—the prohibition against policy rescissions after subscribers become sick and the requirement that insurers spend 85 percent of premium dollars on medical services.

Another implementation action involved sending guidance to small businesses to advise them of the health care tax credits available in 2010 and subsequent years. HHS also planned to distribute the $250 Medicare rebate checks to seniors. In addition, HHS reached out to states to set up high-risk insurance pools to help provide affordable health insurance coverage to adults who are uninsured because of preexisting conditions. The ACA allows states to choose whether to participate in the program, and if a state does not set up a state pool, people from that state can apply for coverage in a federal high-risk pool. As of May 2010, thirty states had chosen to operate their own insurance pools, while eighteen chose to use the federal pool for their eligible citizens.

The administration took another significant step in July 2010, when the president appointed Harvard professor and health care expert Don Berwick to head the Center for Medicaid and Medicare Services—an agency within HHS charged with running Medicare and Medicaid. Obama made the appointment while the Senate was in recess (when appointments do not require a Senate vote) because Senate Republicans had promised to stall the nomination indefinitely. Berwick is widely respected as an advocate for patient-centered health care, but some Republicans said he was too supportive of the single-payer, British model of health care, which they claim embraces rationing of health care.

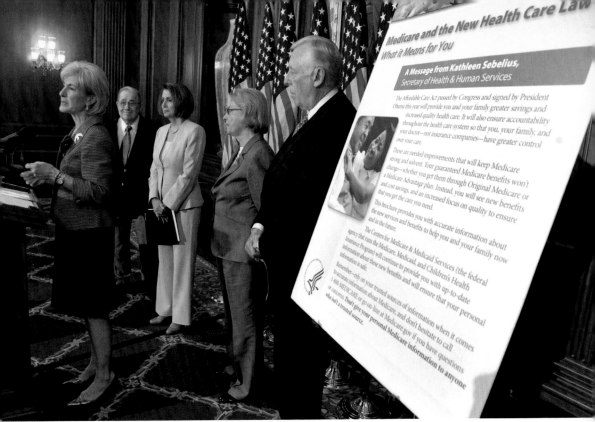

Health and human services secretary Kathleen Sebelius, accompanied by Democratic congressional leaders, holds a press conference in May 2010 to discuss the benefits and misconceptions of the Affordable Care Act.

The federal government next focused on engaging the public and getting out a positive message about the benefits of the ACA. Sebelius met with various groups to explain the ACA and answer questions, and HHS set up a new website called HealthCare .gov filled with news and information about the new law, including a Patients' Bill of Rights—an explanation of the new ACA regulations that apply to health coverage as of September 23, 2010. As part of a $125 million public relations campaign, the administration also rolled out a television ad featuring TV star Andy Griffith discussing how the ACA will strengthen health care for seniors.

Effects of Health Care Reform on Access to Health Care

Despite the administration's efforts to portray the ACA as a vast improvement for U.S. health care, however, analysts looking at the details of the law raised concerns about the law's long-term effects on access to health care. On the plus side, most health care experts agree that the ACA will provide better access to health care for many Americans since it will mandate health insurance coverage for millions of the uninsured, expand Medicaid to cover an additional 16 million lower-income people, and allow parents to keep their children on their policies until age twenty-six.

CONTROLLING HEALTH CARE COSTS

"At the end of the day, [the Affordable Care Act] . . . is largely about the worthy goal of expanding access to coverage, rather than the pressing imperative of addressing explosive health care costs. . . . Therefore, . . . the law is likely worse than doing nothing at all." —U.S. Chamber of Commerce, a business federation representing the interests of more than 3 million U.S. businesses of all sizes, sectors, and regions, as well as state and local chambers and industry associations.

U.S. Chamber of Commerce, "Critical Issues in the Patient and Affordable Care Act." www.uschamber.com/assets/labor/100426_critical_employer_issues_ppaca.pdf.

However, critics say the ACA will still leave many people with restricted access to care. Many commentators argue that the ACA will allow younger, healthier people to game the system by opting out of insurance coverage (by paying small fines)— until they get sick, when they can apply for coverage without fear of being denied for a preexisting condition. As a *San Diego Union-Tribune* editorial opines: "With fines for noncompliance being relatively small and with insurers compelled to provide coverage to anyone who applies, individuals have a financial incentive to not get insurance until a health issue makes it necessary."[48] Largely because of this dynamic, John Geyman, a professor of family medicine at the University of Washington School of Medicine, predicts that as of 2019 as many as 23 million people could still be uninsured. Millions more, he says, will be underinsured for various reasons. For example, he thinks that many people will not be able to afford the insurance offered in the high-risk insurance exchanges, and that the new federal high-risk pool will be inadequate to meet the needs of the many people who will apply there for coverage. Geyman concludes, "Despite the hype we hear about "near-universal" access just down the road . . . access to care will remain inadequate for much of the population."[49]

Other commentators worry that even currently insured people could lose coverage since the ACA allows employers to pay a penalty instead of providing health insurance. In fact, news reports have already surfaced suggesting that some large companies might dump health care coverage for their employees entirely since it will be cheaper to simply pay the penalty. Former House speaker Newt Gingrich has even predicted that "the employer-based system will collapse" due to this provision.[50]

Effects of Health Care Reform on the Quality of Health Care

Similarly, while the ACA does include a number of provisions that will likely improve the quality of health care, the law has also been criticized in this area. The ACA has been praised, on the one hand, for eliminating various insurance industry abuses. In addition, according to new rules issued by the government, the ACA will require insurers to pay the full cost of preventive medical services that get an "A" or "B" recommendation from the U.S. Preventive Services Task Force, a volunteer group made up of primary care and public health experts. According to reporter Robert Pear of the *New York Times*, "The new requirements promise significant benefits for consumers. . . . The rules will eliminate co-payments, deductibles and other charges for blood pressure; diabetes and cholesterol tests; many cancer screenings; routine vaccinations; prenatal care; and regular wellness visits for infants and children."[51]

Moreover, ACA supporters point out that the new law contains a number of provisions directly geared toward improving the quality and efficiency of the health care system. In Medicare, for example, incentives will be provided to hospitals that meet performance standards for care and efficient use of resources. In addition, Medicare soon will pay a bonus to primary

The Massachusetts Health Care Reforms

Many commentators say the Affordable Care Act (ACA) closely resembles health care reforms enacted in 2006 by the state of Massachusetts. Both the state program and the ACA, for example, require most people to have health insurance, with fines for noncompliance and subsidies for those too young to qualify for Medicare but too poor to afford private insurance. Like the ACA, the state program also requires insurers to accept anyone who applies, prohibiting exclusions for pre-existing conditions. In Massachusetts, these reforms expanded insurance coverage for the nonelderly population (from 87.5 percent in 2006 to 95.2 percent by 2009) and gave people greater access to medical services with lower out-of-pocket costs. However, critics say that the Massachusetts reforms did little to control soaring health care costs. Also, because fines were set low, critics claim the Massachusetts law encourages people to wait until they are sick before purchasing health insurance—a flaw that causes insurance premiums to be higher than if all healthy people were included in the insurance pool. In response to rising insurance rates, the state rejected premium hikes for small employers, later negotiating for smaller increases. Critics say that both the Massachusetts law and the ACA avoid effective cost control measures, such as curbing incomes of doctors and other providers or limiting people's choice of doctors, because such measures are politically unpopular.

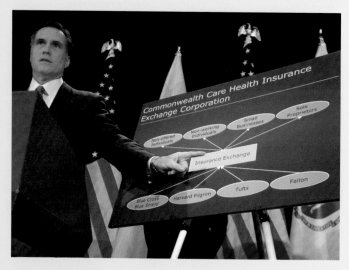

In April 2005 Massachusetts governor Mitt Romney spoke about the state's health care reform bill, which he says will cover virtually all Massachusetts residents by 2009.

care doctors for certain procedures, and funding will be made available to encourage training for certain primary care physicians. A central part of this strategy, too, is a plan to measure the performance of medical providers so that changes can be made in the future to enhance the quality of care.

Yet critics are not convinced that the ACA will do enough to improve quality. They point out that many people already covered by health insurance plans will not benefit from some of the ACA's insurance reforms because health insurance plans that existed as of the March 23, 2010, date of the ACA's enactment will be "grandfathered"—that is, exempted. According to rules issued by HHS on June 14, 2010, for example, reforms requiring coverage of preventive care, coverage of emergency medical services without prior authorization, coverage of essential health benefits, and new appeal procedures will not be applied to grandfathered plans. The HHS regulations, however, provide that plans will lose their grandfathered status if significant changes are made to the plan that reduce benefits or increase costs to participants. According to some analysts, this will mean that most existing plans will eventually lose their grandfathered status and be brought into the fold of health care reform.

Yet critics worry that insurance companies will still find other ways to game the new law to enhance profits at the expense of patient care. As *Mother Jones* blogger Kevin Drum explains,

> Starting in 2014 insurance companies will no longer be allowed to discriminate against people with preexisting conditions. They'll have to take all comers for (almost) the same price, regardless of how healthy they are. The incentive here is obvious: within the confines of the law, insurance companies will do their best to lure the healthiest patients into their programs and convince the sickest ones to switch.[52]

At the other end of the political spectrum, conservatives argue that the biggest threat to quality care is that ACA will give the federal government too much control over medical providers. They point to the ACA's plan to cut Medicare reimbursements to providers and use comparative effectiveness research—that is, research about which medical protocols are the most effective—in making Medicare reimbursement decisions. The libertarian Cato Institute's Michael Tanner argues that the end result of this increased government meddling in medical decisions will be a shortage of physicians. As Tanner explains,

> The United States already faces a potential shortage of physicians, especially primary-care physicians and certain specialties such as geriatric care. Some estimates suggest we will face a shortage of more than 150,000 physicians in the next 15 years. The legislation itself could exacerbate this trend. . . . Indeed, one survey found that 45 percent of physicians would at least consider the possibility of quitting as a result of this health care legislation.[53]

A loss of physicians, Tanner says, would be especially problematic now, because the ACA's expansion of coverage will increase the demand for health care.

Health Care Reform and Health Care Costs

Whether the ACA will fulfill another key goal of reform—controlling health care costs of individuals, businesses, and the government—is probably the most hotly debated question following its passage. One area of dispute is the cost of the ACA itself. The independent research agency the Congressional Budget Office (CBO) estimates that the ACA will cost $940 billion over ten years, but because various tax increases and spending cuts offset new spending programs, the CBO estimates the law will actually reduce the national deficit by $143 billion during that period. As *Washington Post* reporter Ezra Klein explains, this means "the ACA wipes out about a quarter to a third of our long-term deficit."[54] However, critics dispute these figures. According to Tanner's analysis, for example, "The legislation will cost far more than advertised, more than $2.7 trillion over 10 years of full implementation, and will add $352 billion to the national debt over that period."[55]

Another issue is the effect the ACA will have on rapidly rising costs of health insurance for employers and individuals. Many commentators have argued that the ACA's addition of new mandated insurance benefits will cause insurance rates to continue to rise even faster than before health reform because insurers will be paying out more in claims. As Tanner concludes: "Most American workers and businesses will see little or no change in their skyrocketing insurance costs, while millions of others, including younger and healthier workers and those who buy insurance on their own through the non-group market will actually see their premiums go up faster as a result of this legislation."[56] In fact, the CBO does project that the average family health insurance premium, at least for individual policies, could increase to $15,200 by 2016—about a 14 percent increase from the current average of $13,100. The Obama administration has promised to require insurers to justify unreasonable premium increases and to enforce the ACA requirement that insurers spend at least 80 percent of premium dollars on medical services, but, as Pear warns, "some insurers may curtail sales to individuals or small businesses if they find the requirements too difficult to meet."[57]

Congressional Budget Office officials Glenn Hackbart, left, and Doug Elmendorf informed Congress that the Affordable Care Act would actually reduce the national deficit by $143 billion in ten years.

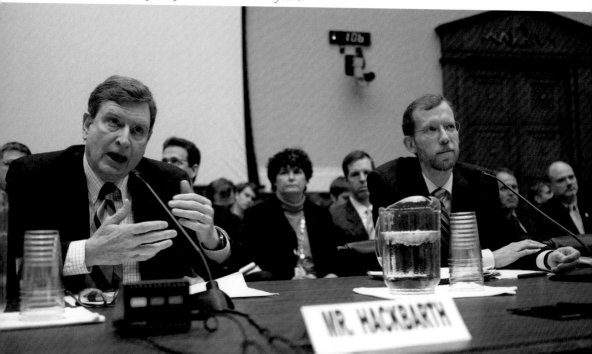

Critics of the ACA also complain that it embodies huge tax increases—according to some projections, a total of $669 billion between now and 2019. One of the main taxes in the ACA is the tax on high-premium "Cadillac" plans, both those provided by employers and plans purchased by individuals—basically a tax on 40 percent of the premium amount above $10,200 for individual coverage (above $27,500 for family coverage). Other taxes are levied on drug manufacturers, health insurance companies, and medical device manufacturers. In addition, as noted earlier, the ACA imposes penalties on large employers who fail to provide basic health insurance for employees and on individuals who fail to purchase insurance. By targeting businesses and consumers, according to conservatives, the taxes will retard economic growth and mandate the unfair redistribution of wealth from the rich to the poor. The taxes on providers, they contend, will simply be passed on to consumers through higher health care costs.

RATIONING

"Rising costs will make rationing in one form or another inevitable in every country, including the United States." —Karen Dillon and Steve Prokesch, editors for the *Harvard Business Review*.

Karen Dillon and Steve Prokesch, "Global Challenges in Health Care: Is Rationing in Our Future?" *Harvard Business Review*, April 5, 2010. http://blogs.hbr.org/cs/2010/04/global_challenges_in_health_ca.html?cm_mmc=npv-_-DAILY_ALERT-_-AWEBER-_-DATE.

ACA supporters, on the other hand, defend the CBO budget numbers and note the ACA's numerous cost control provisions. For example, besides the various cost-saving changes in Medicare and Medicaid, the ACA includes measures against fraud and abuse, paperwork reductions, incentives for the use of generic drugs, and elimination of subsidies for the Medicare Advantage program. The Cadillac tax, proponents say, provides incentives for employers and insurers to develop more cost-effective plans. In addition, the ACA includes provisions geared toward changing the way health care is delivered to make it more coordinated and efficient. In this category are provisions to encourage the use of electronic records, incentives to force hospitals to adopt practices to reduce their rates of hospital-acquired infections, and numerous pilot and demonstration projects to test cost-control ideas. Another hope is that the ACA-mandated health insurance exchanges will spur competition among insurers and lead to more affordable insurance plans. As health care experts Peter R. Orszag and Ezekiel J. Emanuel argue:

> [The ACA] puts into place virtually every cost-control reform proposed by physicians, economists, and health policy experts and includes the means for these reforms to be assessed quickly and scaled up if they're successful. By enacting a broad portfolio of changes, the ACA provides the best assurance that effective change will occur. Moreover, by taking a multifaceted approach that includes hard savings plus the mechanisms for creating a dynamic health care system, it enables physicians, hospitals, and other providers to consistently improve outcomes, boost quality, and reduce costs as health care evolves.[58]

Senator Bernie Sanders (I-Vt), speaks for organized labor to the press about labor's opposition to taxing high-value health insurance plans, the so-called Cadillac tax.

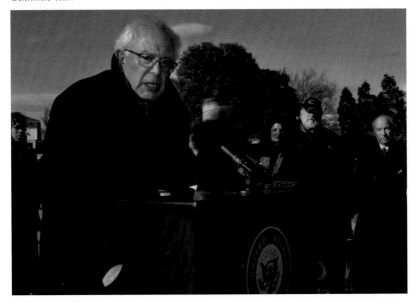

Future Innovations in Health Care

Given the serious debates about the impact ACA will have on U.S. health care, as well as the act's complexity, years will likely pass before Americans can fairly judge whether the reforms are truly helpful. Meanwhile, many health experts hope the assessment and pilot programs contained in the law may reveal better ways of doing things that will encourage future health care reforms. For example, one key pilot program scheduled for implementation by January 2013 tests a new way to pay for medical services. Instead of the traditional fee-for-service system, in which medical providers are paid for each patient visit or service, the pilot program will use bundled payments—that is, lump sum or grouped payments—to encourage doctors and hospitals to coordinate care and share accountability for each hospital stay. Many health experts argue that moving away from the fee-for-service payment system that pays for quantity of care rather than quality is the only way to hold down health care costs. If this pilot program works, it could become a model for Medicare as well as private sector health care.

Another part of the ACA's scheme is the new Center for Medicare and Medicaid Innovation, which will encourage communities and local health systems to experiment with ways to deliver better care at lower costs. The center will be responsible for developing various reform models—such as patient-centered medical homes, promotion of care coordination through salary-based payments to physicians, community-based health teams, and use of information technology to coordinate care for the chronically ill—which will be tested in local communities. As surgeon and health care writer Atul Gawande explains, "In large part, it entrusts the task of devising cost-saving health-care innovation to communities like Boise and Boston and Buffalo, rather than to the drug and device companies and the public and private insurers that have failed to do so. . . . Far from being a government takeover, it counts on local communities and clinicians for success."[59]

Some commentators, however, predict that the ultimate goal of the ACA is to move toward a national, government-run health care system similar to those in Europe. This could occur, analysts say, because the ACA's heavy regulation of insurers could

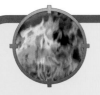

The Future of Health Care Technology

Studies comparing the United States with other countries have found that the U.S. health care system lags behind the rest of the developed world in embracing information technology. In fact, according to the independent research agency the Congressional Budget Office (CBO), only 12 percent of America's physicians and 11 percent of its hospitals had adopted computerized record keeping systems as of 2006. Instead, most U.S. doctors and medical providers use a patchwork of paper systems for keeping patient records, billing, and scheduling. This system is not only inefficient it also results in high administration costs that are passed along to consumers and contribute to rising health care costs. Recent reforms and legislation therefore have sought to address these deficiencies. In February 2009, for example, the American Recovery and Reinvestment Act—President Obama's economic stimulus package—included about $19 billion to expand the use of health information technology. This investment, supporters say, will be used to implement a nationwide electronic medical records (EMR) system, among other technologies—a radical improvement that the CBO estimates could save $7 billion in the first five years. EMR is also expected to improve care for patients. A basic EMR system will give doctors a wealth of patient information, which should help them make faster and more accurate diagnoses and will allow patients to more easily schedule a visit, get reminders about annual check-ups and appointments, and review lab test results. The 2010 Affordable Care Act (ACA) attempts to build on this effort by including additional incentives for the efficient organization and delivery of health care.

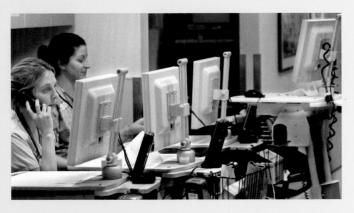

Children's Hospital in Pittsburgh, Pennsylvania, took seven years and $10 million in equipment purchases to create a paperless campus. By going paperless, health care institutions will save big money.

drive up the costs of health insurance and thereby create public support for a national health insurance program. As Gingrich suggests, "When employees realize the high costs of the health care exchanges, they will demand a nationalized health care system."[60] Still others fear that the ACA will strengthen the private insurance system. As single-payer supporter Rob Stone argues: "The new legislation hands over $350 billion in government subsidies to the private insurers while mandating consumers to buy the industry's shoddy products. That, combined with a lack of price controls means the ACA could prove to be a bonanza for the corporate stakeholders in the medical-industrial complex."[61]

A STARTING POINT FOR HEALTH CARE REFORM

"PPACA is the start of a decades long process of remaking the health care system in the United States." —Wallis S. Stromberg, a Denver, Colorado, attorney who practices health care law, representing physicians, hospitals, provider networks, and other health care providers.

Wallis S. Stromberg, "PPACA—the Starting Point for Reform," DGS Health Law Blog, May 20, 2010. www.dgshealthlaw.com/articles/health-care-reform.

The reality is that no one knows at this point exactly what the future ramifications of the ACA will be or what additional reforms might be considered in the future. In the meantime, each side in the health care debate will continue to push its agenda. How the U.S. health care system will be affected by all of these forces will likely be revealed over the course of months, years, and quite possibly decades.

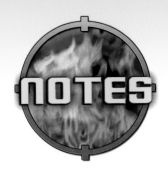

Introduction: The Uninsured in America

1. Quoted in Steven Reinberg, *U.S. Health Care Ranks Low Among Developed Nations: Report*, Center for Advanced Medicine and Clinical Research, June 23, 2010. www.drbuttar .com/blog/?p=1229.
2. Robert Wood Johnson Foundation, "Quick Facts on the Uninsured," Cover the Uninsured, 2009. http://covertheun insured.org/content/quick-facts-uninsured.
3. Quoted in Jonathan Cohn, "When You Are Denied Health Insurance Benefits," MSNBC, October 6, 2008. www.ms nbc.msn.com/id/26664727/ns/health-health_care/page/2.

Chapter 1: America's Health Care System

4. Jonathan Cohn, *Sick: The Untold Story of America's Health Care Crisis*. New York: HarperCollins, 2007, p. 6.
5. Cohn, *Sick*, p. 31.
6. Quoted in Cohn, *Sick*, p. 35.
7. Arnold S. Relman, *A Second Opinion: Rescuing America's Health Care*. New York: Public Affairs, 2007, pp. 51–52.
8. Tom Daschle, *Critical: What We Can Do About the Health Care Crisis*. New York: St. Martin's, 2008, p. 62.
9. Marian E. Gornick, Joan L. Warren, Paul W. Eggers, James D. Lubitz, Nancy De Lew, Margaret H. Davis, and Barbara S. Cooper, "Thirty Years of Medicare: Impact on the Covered Population," *Health Care Financing Review*, vol. 18, no. 2, Winter 1996, p. 179. www.ssa.gov/history/pdf/ThirtyYears Population.pdf.
10. Daschle, *Critical*, p. 63.
11. Relman, *A Second Opinion*, p. 44.

12. Corinne Mitchell, "The History of HMOs," *Ezine Articles*, 2010. http://ezinearticles.com/?The-History-of-HMO-Plans& id=2113007.

Chapter 2: The Debate About Health Care Reform

13. Karen S. Palmer, "A Brief History: Universal Health Care Efforts in the US," Physicians for a National Health Program, Spring 1999. www.pnhp.org/facts/a_brief_history_universal_ health_care_efforts_in_the_us.php?page=all.

14. Palmer, "A Brief History."

15. George W. Bush, "THE 2004 CAMPAIGN; Transcript of Debate Between Bush and Kerry, with Domestic Policy the Topic," *New York Times*, October 14, 2004. http://query.ny times.com/gst/fullpage.html?res=9C02EFDF163AF937A25 753C1A9629C8B63&sec=&spon=&pagewanted=6.

16. Karl Rove, "ObamaCare Isn't Inevitable," *Wall Street Journal*, June 25, 2009. http://online.wsj.com/article/SB124588 632634150501.html.

17. Rove, "ObamaCare Isn't Inevitable."

18. Daschle, *Critical*, p. 3.

19. David U. Himmelstein, Deborah Thorne, Elizabeth Warren, and Steffie Woolhandler, "Medical Bankruptcy in the United States, 2007: Results of a National Study," *American Journal of Medicine*, 2009. http://healthcare.procon.org/sourcefiles/ HimmelsteinMedicalBankruptcy2007.pdf.

20. George P. Shultz and John B. Shoven, *Putting Our House in Order: A Guide to Social Security and Health Care Reform*. New York: W.W. Norton, 2008, p. 138.

21. Relman, *A Second Opinion*, pp. 105–6.

22. Cynthia Tucker, "Shouting, Stomping Won't Obscure Need for Reform," Appealdemocrat.com, August 9, 2009. www .appeal-democrat.com/articles/health-85291-care-consum ers.html.

23. Eric Kimbuende, Usha Ranji, Janet Lundy, and Alina Salganicoff, "Health Care Costs," Kaiseredu.com, March 2010. www.kaiseredu.org/topics_im.asp?imID=1&parentID=61 &id=358.

24. Arnold S. Relman, "Waiting for the Health Reform We Really Need," *Tikkun*, September 24, 2009. www.tikkun.org/article.php/20090924083334396.

25. Stan Lebowitz, "Policy Analysis: Why Health Care Costs Too Much," Cato Institute, June 23, 1994. www.cato.org/pubs/pas/pa211.html.

Chapter 3: Health Care Systems in Other Countries

26. National Institute of Medicine, "Insuring America's Health: Principles and Recommendations," January 13, 2004. www.iom.edu/Reports/2004/Insuring-Americas-Health-Principles-and-Recommendations.aspx.

27. Palmer, "A Brief History."

28. T.R. Reid, *The Healing of America: The Global Quest for Better, Cheaper, and Fairer Health Care*. New York: Penguin, 2009, p. 19.

29. Richard Knox, "Most Patients Happy with German Health Care," National Public Radio, August 3, 2010. www.npr.org/templates/story/story.php?storyId=91971406.

30. Quoted in Reid, *The Healing of America*, p. 76.

31. Reid, *The Healing of America*, p. 103.

32. *Bloomberg Businessweek*, "The French Lesson in Health Care," July 9, 2007. www.businessweek.com/magazine/content/07_28/b4042070.htm.

33. World Health Organization, "World Health Organization Assesses the World's Health Systems," 2000. www.who.int/whr/2000/media_centre/press_release/en.

34. Karen David, Cathy Schoen, and Kristof Stremikis, "Mirror, Mirror on the Wall: How the Performance of the U.S. Health Care System Compares Internationally," Commonwealth Fund, June 2010. www.commonwealthfund.org/~/media/Files/Publications/Fund%20Report/2010/Jun/1400_Davis_Mirror_Mirror_on_the_wall_2010.pdf.

35. Robert Moffit, Philippe Manière, David Green, Paul Belien, Johan Hjertqvist, and Friedrich Breyer, "Perspectives on the European Health Care Systems: Some Lessons for America," Heritage Foundation, July 9, 2001. www.heritage.org/

Research/Lecture/Perspectives-on-the-European-Health-Care-Systems.

Chapter 4: The Patient Protection and Affordable Care Act

36. Ted Kennedy, "Ted Kennedy's Obama Endorsement— Transcript," Wordpress.com, January 28, 2008. http://the kennedys.wordpress.com/2008/01/29/ted-kennedys-obama-endorsement-transcript.

37. Barack Obama, "Obama's Health Care Speech to Congress," *New York Times*, September 9, 2009. www.ny times.com/2009/09/10/us/politics/10obama.text.html?page wanted=1&_r=2.

38. Quoted in Sheryl Gay Stolberg and Robert Pear, "Obama Signs Health Care Overhaul Bill, with a Flourish," *New York Times*, March 23, 2010. www.nytimes.com/2010/03/24/health/policy/24health.html.

39. Jim Giles, "Socialised Medicine and Death Panels: Business as Usual," *New Scientist*, August 14, 2009. www.new scientist.com/blogs/shortsharpscience/2009/08/socialised-medicine-and-death.html.

40. Quoted in Laura Meckler, "Health-Care Battle Set to Focus on Public Plan," *Wall Street Journal*, March 24, 2009. http://online .wsj.com/article/NA_WSJ_PUB:SB123785156695519283 .html.

41. Robert Reich, "New Health Care Bill: Biggest Change Since Medicare?" *Christian Science Monitor*, March 22, 2010. www .csmonitor.com/Money/Robert-Reich-s-Blog/2010/0322/New-health-care-bill-Biggest-change-since-Medicare.

42. David Leonhardt, "In Health Bill, Obama Attacks Wealth Inequality," *New York Times*, March 23, 2010. www.nytimes .com/2010/03/24/business/24leonhardt.html.

43. Dennis Kucinich, John Conyers, and Bernie Sanders, statement dated July 29, 2010. http://sanders.senate.gov/graphics/buzz/single_payer_ltr.pdf.

44. Kevin Hassett, "Obamacare Only Looks Worse upon Further Review," August 1, 2010. www.bloomberg.com/news/

2010-08-02/obamacare-only-looks-worse-upon-further-review-kevin-hassett.html.

45. Barack Obama, "Remarks by the President on the Affordable Care Act and the New Patients' Bill of Rights," White House, June 22, 2010. www.whitehouse.gov/the-press-office/re marks-president-affordable-care-act-and-new-patients-bill-rights.

Chapter 5: The Future of U.S. Health Care

46. Quoted in *Huffington Post*, "Jim DeMint: Health Care Bill 'Must Be Repealed,' Plans to Introduce Legislation," March 22, 2010. www.huffingtonpost.com/2010/03/22/jim-de mint-health-care-bi_n_508060.html.

47. Maggie Mahar, "A Reply to the Cato Institute's Report on Healthcare Reform—Part 1," Health Beat, July 16, 2010. www.healthbeatblog.com/2010/07/a-reply-to-the-cato-in stitutes-report-on-healthcare-reform-part-1-.html.

48. *San Diego Union-Tribune*, "U-T Editorial: Fix Health Law's Flaws: Results in Massachusetts Show System Will Be Gamed," July 11, 2010. www.sduniontribune.com/ news/2010/jul/11/u-t-editorial-fix-health-laws-flaws.

49. John Geyman, "Hijacked: Stolen Health Reform III: How Much Will Access to Care Be Expanded?" Physicians for a National Health Program, July 15, 2010. http://pnhp.org/ blog/2010/07/15/hijacked-stolen-health-reform-iii-how-much-will-access-to-care-be-expanded.

50. Quoted in Rob Stone, "Progressives and Conservatives Agree: Single Payer Healthcare Is Inevitable," *Huffington Post,* August 10, 2010. www.huffingtonpost.com/rob-stone-md/progressives-and-conserva_b_676488.html.

51. Robert Pear, "Health Plans Must Provide Some Tests at No Cost," *New York Times*, July 14, 2010. www.ny times.com/2010/07/15/health/policy/15health.html?_ r=3&emc=tnt&tntemail0=y.

52. Kevin Drum, "Will Insurance Companies Game the ACA?" *Mother Jones*, August 16, 2010. http://motherjones.com/ kevin-drum/2010/08/will-insurance-companies-game-aca.

53. Michael Tanner, "Bad Medicine: A Guide to the Real Costs and Consequences of the New Health Care Law," Cato Institute, 2010. www.cato.org/pubs/wtpapers/BadMedicineWP .pdf.

54. Ezra Klein, "OMB, ACA, CBO and the Deficit," *Washington Post*, July 8, 2010. http://voices.washingtonpost.com/ ezra-klein/2010/07/omb_aca_cbo_and_the_deficit.html.

55. Tanner, "Bad Medicine."

56. Tanner, "Bad Medicine."

57. Robert Pear, "Covering New Ground in Health System Shift," *New York Times*, August 2, 2010. www.nytimes .com/2010/08/03/health/policy/03insurance.html?_r=2&hp.

58. Peter R. Orszag and Ezekiel J. Emanuel, "Health Care Reform and Cost Control," *New England Journal of Medicine*, June 16, 2010. http://healthpolicyandreform.nejm.org/?p=3564.

59. Atul Gawande, "Now What?" *New Yorker*, April 5, 2010. www .newyorker.com/talk/comment/2010/04/05/100405taco_ talk_gawande#ixzz0wuAa1XBd.

60. Quoted in Stone, "Progressives and Conservatives Agree."

61. Stone, "Progressives and Conservatives Agree."

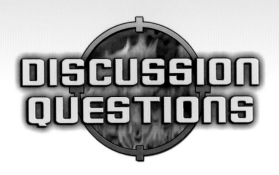

DISCUSSION QUESTIONS

Chapter 1: America's Health Care System

1. How did Blue Cross get started in the health insurance business, according to the author?
2. How did World War II affect the U.S. system of health insurance?
3. What does the concept of "experience rating" have to do with how health insurance coverage is granted in America?
4. What is managed care, as explained in this chapter?

Chapter 2: The Debate About Health Care Reform

1. Which U.S. president helped to enact Medicare/Medicaid in 1965?
2. What was the 1988 Medicare Catastrophic Coverage Act (MCCA), and why was it repealed, according to the author?
3. Describe some pros and cons of the U.S. health care system, as articulated by various participants in the debate about health reform.
4. How do conservatives and progressives differ in their views about the role of government in providing health care for Americans, according to this book?

Chapter 3: Health Care Systems in Other Countries

1. What is the Bismarck model of health care, according to writer T.R. Reid?
2. Describe some of the features of Britain's national health care program, and explain why it might be called a socialized system.
3. Which country's health care system has been ranked number one by the World Health Organization (WHO)?

4. Where does the United States rank in terms of the quality of health care, according to the World Health Organization?

Chapter 4: The Patient Protection and Affordable Care Act

1. When was the Patient Protection and Affordable Care Act (PPACA), also more simply called the Affordable Care Act (ACA), enacted?

2. Describe the debate in Congress over the "public option" and state whether this feature was included in the final legislation.

3. Name some of the health insurance company practices changed by the Affordable Care Act.

4. Why do many Republicans and conservatives dislike the Affordable Care Act, according to this book?

Chapter 5: The Future of U.S. Health Care

1. What is the main claim in the state lawsuits filed in opposition to the Affordable Care Act, according to the author?

2. What is the Patients' Bill of Rights, as explained in this book?

3. What is the "Cadillac tax?"

4. Do you think that the Affordable Care Act will improve health care in the United States? Why or why not?

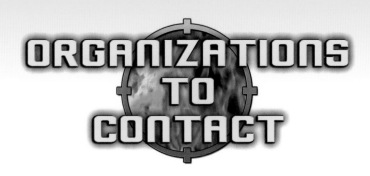

ORGANIZATIONS TO CONTACT

American Medical Association (AMA)
515 N. State St.
Chicago, IL 60654
phone: (800) 621-8335
website: www.ama-assn.org

The American Medical Association is the largest medical association of physicians in the nation. It represents physicians from every state and specialty and works to promote the art and science of medicine and the betterment of public health. The AMA supports meaningful health system reform, and its website contains information, analysis, and articles for physicians and patients about the AMA's position on reform and the impact of the 2010 health care reform law.

The Campaign for an American Solution
phone: (800) 289-1136
e-mail: info@americanhealthsolution.org
website: www.americanhealthsolution.org

The Campaign for an American Solution is a nonpartisan, educational initiative of America's Health Insurance Plans (AHIP), the national trade association for the health insurance industry. The mission of the initiative is to build support for health care reforms favored by insurance companies. The website is a source of information about the industry's views on health care reform, and it contains documents such as position statements, congressional testimony, and links to studies on health care costs.

Center on Budget and Policy Priorities
820 First St. NE, Ste. 510
Washington, DC 20002
phone: (202) 408-1080

fax: (202) 408-1056
e-mail: center@cbpp.org
website: www.cbpp.org

The Center on Budget and Policy Priorities is a policy research organization that works at federal and state levels on fiscal policy and public programs that affect low- and moderate-income families and individuals. The center conducts research and analysis to help shape public debates over proposed budget and tax policies and to help ensure that policy makers consider the needs of low-income families and individuals in these debates. One of the group's main areas of research is health care, and this section of its website contains numerous articles, analyses, and other publications about health care reform, the impact of the 2010 health care law, and other health issues.

Commonwealth Fund
One E. Seventy-fifth St.
New York, NY 10021
phone: (212) 606-3800
fax: (212) 606-3500
website: www.commonwealthfund.org

The Commonwealth Fund is a private foundation that promotes health care reform to achieve better access, improved quality, and greater efficiency, particularly for low-income people, the uninsured, minority Americans, young children, and elderly adults. The fund carries out this mandate by supporting independent research on health care issues and making grants to improve health care practice and policy. The fund produces more than one hundred free publications a year, including several newsletters (such as the *Commonwealth Fund Connection*) and an online *Annual Report*. Recent publications include "Achieving the Vision: Payment Reform" and "Why the Nation Needs a Policy Push on Patient-Centered Health Care."

Institute of Medicine (IOM)
500 Fifth St. NW
Washington, DC 20001
phone: (202) 334-2352

e-mail: iomwww@nas.edu
website: www.iom.edu.

The Institute of Medicine is an independent, nonprofit organization that works outside government to provide unbiased and authoritative advice to decision makers and the public. Established in 1970, the IOM is the health arm of the National Academy of Sciences, which was chartered under President Abraham Lincoln in 1863 to provide advice to the nation about various sciences. The IOM studies health issues, often as a mandate from Congress or as requested by federal agencies and independent organizations, and prepares reports of its findings (available on its website). The IOM also convenes a series of forums, roundtables, and standing committees, as well as other activities, to facilitate discussion, discovery, and critical, cross-disciplinary thinking.

Kaiser Family Foundation—Health Care Reform
2400 Sand Hill Rd.
Menlo Park, CA 94025
phone: (650) 854-9400
fax: (650) 854-4800
website: http://healthreform.kff.org

The Kaiser Family Foundation is a nonprofit privately operating foundation focusing on the major health care issues facing the United States, as well as the U.S. role in global health policy. Unlike grant-making foundations, Kaiser develops and runs its own research and communications programs, sometimes in partnership with other nonprofit research organizations or major media companies. The foundation serves as a nonpartisan source of facts, information, and analysis about health care reform for policy makers, the media, the health care community, and the public. Its website contains a wide range of information, including analyses of the new health care law, issue briefs about health care matters, results of public opinion polls, and congressional testimony.

Physicians for a National Health Program (PNHP)
29 E. Madison St., Ste. 602
Chicago, IL 60602

phone: (312) 782-6006
fax: (312) 782-6007
e-mail: info@pnhp.org

Physicians for a National Health Program is a single-issue organization that advocates for a universal, comprehensive, single-payer national health program. With more than seventeen thousand members and chapters across the United States, the group seeks to educate physicians and other health professionals about the benefits of a single-payer system—including fewer administrative costs and affording health insurance for the 46 million Americans who have none. The PNHP website is a good source for articles about health reform, and the group also publishes a newsletter (for members only), a blog, and press releases.

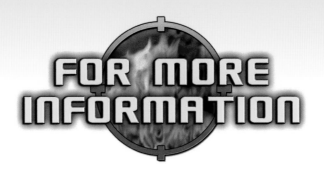

Books

Donald L. Barlett and James B. Steele, *Critical Condition: How Health Care in America Became Big Business—and Bad Medicine.* New York: Broadway Books, 2005. A thoroughly researched indictment of the U.S. health care system, which the authors claim is leaving 44 million Americans without insurance.

David Blumenthal and James Morone, *Heart of Power: Health and Politics in the Oval Office.* Berkeley and Los Angeles: University of California Press, 2009. A history of American health care policy and an investigation of U.S. presidents' attitudes toward the issue.

David Broder and Haynes Johnson, *The System: The American Way of Politics at the Breaking Point.* New York: Back Bay, 1997. An in-depth study of the failure of the Clinton health care reform plan.

Michael F. Cannon, *Healthy Competition: What's Holding Back Health Care and How to Free It, 2nd ed.* Washington, DC: Cato Institute, 2007. An argument against government-controlled health care.

Jonathan Cohn, *Sick: The Untold Story of America's Health Care Crisis—and the People Who Paid the Price.* New York: Harper-Perennial, 2008. An argument for a universal, single-payer health care system regulated by the government, with compelling stories of patients who have suffered health care crises.

Melissa Cox, Henry J. Aaron, and William B. Schwartz, *Can We Say No? The Challenge of Rationing Health Care.* Washington, DC: Brookings Institution, 2005. An argument for sensible health care rationing, based on a review of Great Britain's experiences.

Stephen M. Davidson, *Still Broken: Understanding the U.S. Health Care System.* Palo Alto, CA: Stanford Business Books, 2010. A thorough review of the problems in today's health care, and a proposal for overhauling our system, offering six elements that should be included in any plan for change.

Howard Dean, Igor Volsky, and Faiz Shakir, *Howard Dean's Prescription for Real Healthcare Reform: How We Can Achieve Affordable Medical Care for Every American and Make Our Jobs Safer*. White River Junction, VT: Chelsea Green, 2009. A case for a public health insurance option as the necessary path for solving the health care crisis in America.

David Gratzer, *The Cure: How Capitalism Can Save American Health Care*. New York: Encounter, 2008. A detailed overview of American health care, and a prescription for saving it using capitalism, without growing government or raising taxes.

Regina Herzlinger, *Who Killed Health Care? America's $2 Trillion Medical Problem—and the Consumer-Driven Cure*. New York: Mcgraw-Hill, 2007. A proposal for market-driven, consumer-oriented health care reform to create a national system that would require individuals to buy health insurance, with help in the form of tax breaks and subsidies.

Steven Jonas, Raymond Goldsteen, and Karen Goldsteen, eds., *An Introduction to the U.S. Health Care System*. New York: Springer, 2007. A concise and balanced description of the U.S. health care system.

Peter Kongstvedt, *Managed Care: What It Is and How It Works*. Sudbury, MA: Jones & Bartlett, 2008. A concise introduction to the history and practices of managed health care systems in America.

Robert H. LeBow and C. Rocky White, *Health Care Meltdown: Confronting the Myths and Fixing Our Failing System*. Chambersburg, PA: Alan C. Hood & Company, 2007. A critical analysis of America's health care system and its failings.

T.R. Reid, *The Healing of America: A Global Quest for Better, Cheaper, and Fairer Health Care*. New York: Penguin, 2009. An exploration of health care systems around the world that criticizes the United States for being the only first world nation that has refused to provide its citizens with universal health care.

Leiyu Shi and Douglas A. Singh, *Essentials of the U.S. Health Care System*. Sudbury, MA: Jones & Bartlett, 2009. A clear and concise examination of the basic structures and operations of the U.S. health care system.

Staff of the *Washington Post, Landmark: The Inside Story of America's New Health Care Law and What It Means for Us All*. Cambridge, MA: Public Affairs, 2010. An examination of President Barack Obama's new health care law and its likely impact on families, doctors, hospitals, health care providers, insurers, and other parts of the health care system.

Periodicals

Atul Gawande, "The Cost Conundrum," *New Yorker*, June 1, 2009.

David Goldhill, "How American Health Care Killed My Father," *Atlantic*, September 2009.

Paul Krugman and Robin Wells, "The Health Care Crisis and What to Do About It," *New York Review of Books*, March 23, 2006.

Phillip Longman, "The Best Care Anywhere," *Washington Monthly*, January 2005.

Theodore Marmor, Jonathan Oberlander, and Joseph White, "The Obama Administration's Options for Health Care Cost Control: Hope Versus Reality," *Annals of Internal Medicine*, April 7, 2009.

Kate Michelman, "A System from Hell," *Nation*, April 8, 2009.

Timothy Noah, "Health Reform: An Online Guide: Links to Everything You Need to Know About the Patient Protection and Affordable Care Act of 2010," *Slate*, May 13, 2010. www.slate.com/id/2220222/pagenum.

———, "A Short History of Health Care," *Slate*, March 13, 2007. www.slate.com/id/2161736.

James Ridgeway, "Meet the Real Death Panels: Should Geezers Like Me Give Up Life-Prolonging Treatments to Cut Health Care Costs?" *Mother Jones*, July/August 2010. http://motherjones.com/politics/2010/07/health-care-rationing-death-panels?page=2.

June Thomas, "The American Way of Dentistry," *Slate*, September/October 2009. www.slate.com/id/2229630.

Karen Tumulty, "Making History: House Passes Health Care Reform," *Time*, March 23, 2010. www.time.com/time/politics/article/0,8599,1973989,00.html.

Websites

Fix Health Care Policy (http://fixhealthcarepolicy.com). A website run by the conservative Heritage Foundation dedicated to opposing President Barack Obama's plan for health care reform and criticizing its implementation.

Healthcare.gov (www.healthcare.gov). A federal government website within the Department of Health and Human Services designed to provide information about the Affordable Care Act, a health care reform law signed into law in March 2010.

Healthcarelawsuit.us (www.healthcarelawsuit.us). A website set up by Florida's Office of the Attorney General to provide information and updates on a lawsuit brought against the Affordable Care Act, a health care reform law signed into law in March 2010.

Institute for America's Future: Health Care for All (http://institute.ourfuture.org/issues/health+care+for+all). A research and education center that advocates for progressive solutions for health care reform.

The New England Journal of Medicine: **Health Care** (http://healthcarereform.nejm.org/?emp=marcom). A website run by an academic medical journal containing expert commentary on many different issues surrounding health care reform.

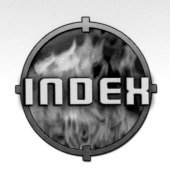

INDEX

A

ACA. *See* Patient Protection and Affordable Care Act

Affordable Care Act (ACA). *See* Patient Protection and Affordable Care Act

Aged
  government health benefits for, 19–22
  See also Medicare

American Association of Labor Legislation (AALL), 27–28

American Federation of Labor, 28

American Journal of Medicine, 35

American Legislative Exchange Council (ALEC), 77

American Medical Association (AMA), 27, 66
  founding of, 11–12

American Recovery and Reinvestment Act (2009), 89

B

Baylor Hospital (Dallas), 13–14

Benson, Craig, 53

Berwick, Don, 78

Beverage, William, 45

Beverage model, 45, 48, 52

Bismarck, Otto von, 44

Bismarck model, 44–45, 46, 52

Blue Cross, 14

Blue Cross/Blue Shield, 16

Brown, Scott, 64

Bush, George W., 32

C

Canada
  health care system in, 52, 54
  prescription drug prices, 53

Carter, Jimmy, 30

CBO (Congressional Budget Office), 68, 89

CCMC (Committee on the Costs of Medical Care), 13

Census Bureau, U.S., 7, 34

Center for Medicaid and Medicare Services, 78

Children's Health Insurance Program, 65

Clinton, Bill, 31–32

Clinton, Hillary, 31, *31,* 60

COBRA (Consolidated Omnibus Budget Reconciliation Act, 1986), 65

Coburn, Tom, 76

Cold War, 30

Committee on Economic Security, 28–29

Committee on the Costs of Medical Care (CCMC), 13

Commonwealth Fund, 56

Comprehensive Health Insurance Act (proposed), 31, 65

Congressional Budget Office (CBO), 68, 89

Consolidated Omnibus Budget Reconciliation Act (COBRA, 1986), 65

Conyers, John, 72

D

Daschle, Tom, 20–21, 34
Demint, Jim, 75–76, 76
Department of Health and
    Human Services, U.S. (HHS),
    78
Developing nations, 45–46
Drugs. *See* Prescription drugs

E

Electronic medical records
    (EMR) system, 42, 70–71,
    87, 89
Elwood, Paul, 23
Emanuel, Ezekiel J., 87
Emergency Medical Treatment
    and Active Labor Act
    (EMTALA, 1986), 65
Employers, 71
EMR (electronic medical
    records) system, 42, 70–71,
    87, 89
EMTALA (Emergency Medical
    Treatment and Active Labor
    Act, 1986), 65
European health care models,
    43–45
    France, 50–52
    Germany, 46–48
    Great Britain, 48–50
    per capita spending in, *vs.* U.S.,
    44

F

Food and Drug Administration,
    U.S. (FDA), 53
Ford, Gerald, 30
France, 50–52
Free clinics, 25
Freedom of Choice in Health
    Care Act (proposed), 77

G

GDP (gross domestic product), 6
    national health expenditures as
        share of, *24*
Germany, 46–48
Geyman, John, 50, 77, 80–81
Gingrich, Newt, 81, 90
Great Britain, National Health
    Service in, 48–50
Great Depression, 28, 29
Gross domestic product (GDP),
    6
    national health expenditures
        as share of, *24*

H

Health care
    arguments on rationing of,
        69
    consumer-driven, 36–37
    future innovations in, 88, 90
    single-payer, 37–38
    universal, 38–39
Health care expenditures, U.S.
    amounts/as share of GDP, *24*
    growth in, 22
    per capital, *vs.* European
        countries, *44*
Health care reform efforts
    as focus of 2008 presidential
        campaign, 60–61
    history of, 27–32
Health insurance
    early programs, 12–14
    employer-based, 15–16
    increasing costs of, 26
    privatization of, 16–19
    rising costs of premiums, 60
Health insurance exchanges, 61,
    63–64, 80–81, 87
Health insurance industry, 40

Health Insurance Portability and
  Accountability Act (HIPAA,
  1996), 65
Health Maintenance Organization
  Act (1973), 23–24
Health maintenance organizations
  (HMOs), 22–24
Health savings accounts (HSAs),
  36
Health Security Act (proposed),
  31–32
Heritage Foundation, 56
HHS (Department of Health and
  Human Services, U.S.), 78
Hurt, Jessica Leanne, 33

I
Ignagni, Karen, 67
Independent Payment Advisory
  Board (IPAB), 69
Institute of Medicine (IOM), 9,
  34–35
IPAB (Independent Payment
  Advisory Board), 69

J
Johnson, Lyndon Baines, 20, *20*,
  30

K
Kaiser Family Foundation, 39–40
Kennedy, Edward, 30, 61, 64, *64*
Kennedy, John F., 20
Kucinich, Dennis, 72

L
Lee, Sheila Jackson, 29

M
Malpractice suits, 42
Managed care, 22–24

Massachusetts, 82
Medicaid, 7, 21
  creation of, 30
  expansion under Patient
    Protection and Affordable
    Care Act, 71
Medicare, 7, 19
  efficiency of, 41
  expansion under Patient
    Protection and Affordable
    Care Act, 71
  expansion under Reagan, 30–31
  parts of, 15
  passage of, 20
Medicare Catastrophic Coverage
  Act (MCCA, 1988), 31
Medicare Modernization Act
  (2003), 65
Moore, Michael, 54, 57

N
National Association of Free
  Clinics, 25
National Labor Relations Board,
  16
Nelson, Ben, 64
Nixon, Richard, 23, 30

O
Obama, Barack, 10, 59, *60*, *63*
  on benefits of Patient Protection
    and Affordable Care Act, 74
  health care reform proposal of,
    62–64
  pledges health care reform, 61
Opinion polls. *See* Surveys
Orszag, Peter R., 87

P
Patient Protection and Affordable
  Care Act (PPACA or ACA,
  2010), 10, 59

criticism of, 71–74
early implementation of
provisions of, 78–79
effects on health care access,
79–81
effects on health care costs,
84–87
effects on health care quality, 81
efforts to repeal, 75–77
reforms in, 68–71
Patients' Bill of Rights, 79
Polls. *See* Surveys
Potter, Wendell, 40, *40*
PPACA. *See* Patient Protection
and Affordable Care Act
Preexisting conditions, 8, 26
coverage under Patient
Protection and Affordable
Care Act, 68–70, 71, 83
high-risk insurance pools for, 78
in HIPAA, 65
Preferred provider organizations
(PPOs), 26
Prescription drugs
Canadian regulation of prices,
53
coverage under Medicare, 65,
70
Price, Tom, 68

R
Race/ethnicity, 8
Reagan, Ronald, 30–31
Reich, Robert, 68
Reid, T.R., 34, 44, 45
Robert Woods Johnson
Foundation, 8

Romney, Mitt, 82
Roosevelt, Franklin D., 28, *28*,
29, 30
Rove, Karl, 32, 34

S
Sanders, Bernie, 72, 87
Sebelius, Kathleen, 61, 78, 79
Shultz, George P., 14, 36
Sicko (film), 54, 57
Social Security Act (1935), 29
State Children's Health Insurance
Program, 7
Surveys
on American's satisfaction with
health care, 55
on Patient Protection and
Affordable Care Act, 74
Switzerland, 58

T
Truman, Harry, 29–30

U
Uninsured, 68
by household income, 9
numbers/characteristics of,
7–8
U.S. Chamber of Commerce, 80
U.S. Pharmaceutical Industry
Report, 32

W
Wagner, Robert F., 29
Weil, Andrew, 41
World Health Organization
(WHO), 34, 54–55

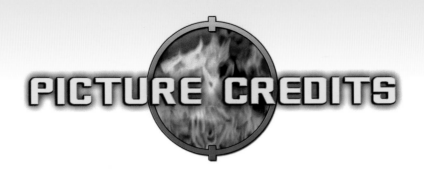

PICTURE CREDITS

Cover: © D. Hurst/Alamy

AP Images, 7, 12, 20, 23, 28, 31, 35, 39, 53, 73, 76, 82, 87, 89

Alexandra Beier/Reuters/Landov, 47

© Bettman/Corbis, 13

Blank Archives/Getty Images, 17

Alexandra Boulat/VII/AP Images, 51

Bill Clark/Roll Call/Getty Images, 72

Kevin Dietsch/UPI/Landov, 65, 79

Dog Eat Dog Films/Weinstein Company/The Kobal Collection/
   The Picture Desk, Inc., 57

Scott J. Ferrell/Congressional Quarterly/Getty Images, 85

Gale/Cengage Learning, 9, 24, 44

© David Levenson/Alamy, 48

Jim Lo Scalzo/EPA/Landov, 25

Phil McCarten/UPI/Landov, 67

Jason Reed/UPI/Landov, 63

Pete Souza/MAI/Landov, 60

Alex Wong/Getty Images, 40

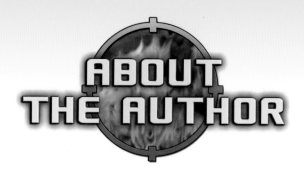

ABOUT THE AUTHOR

Debra A. Miller is a writer and lawyer with a passion for current events, history, and public policy. She began her law career in Washington, D.C., where she worked on legislative, policy, and legal matters in government, public interest, and private law firm positions. She now lives with her husband in Encinitas, California. She has written and edited numerous books and anthologies on historical, political, health, and other topics.